Overview Map Key

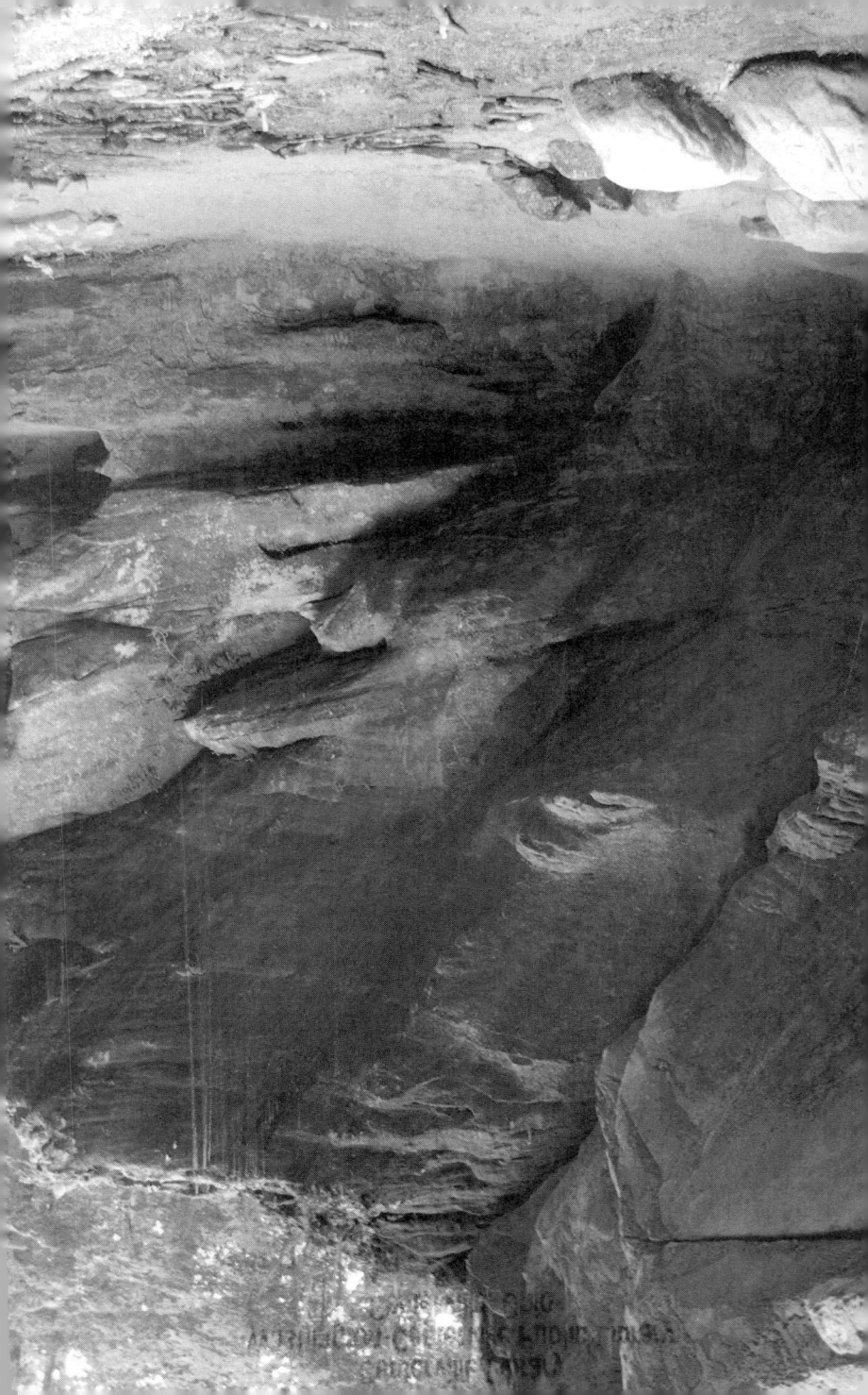

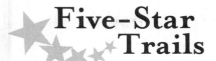

Five-Star Trails

Columbus

Your Guide to the Area's Most Beautiful Hikes

Robert Loewendick

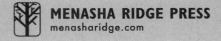

MENASHA RIDGE PRESS
menasharidge.com

Five-Star Trails Columbus
Your Guide to the Area's Most Beautiful Hikes

Copyright © 2013 by Robert Loewendick
All rights reserved
Published by Menasha Ridge Press
Distributed by Publishers Group West
Printed in the United States of America
First edition, first printing

Cover design by Scott McGrew
Frontispiece: Big Lyons Falls at Mohican State Park, page 92
Text design by Annie Long
Cover photographs by Robert Loewendick
All interior photographs by Robert Loewendick
Cartography and elevation profiles by Scott McGrew

CATALOGING-IN-PUBLICATION DATA IS AVAILABLE FROM THE LIBRARY OF CONGRESS.

ISBN 978-0-89732-966-8; eISBN 978-0-89732-976-7

Menasha Ridge Press
P.O. Box 43673
Birmingham, AL 35243
menasharidgepress.com

DISCLAIMER

This book is meant only as a guide to select trails in Columbus, Ohio. This book does not guarantee hiker safety in any way—you hike at your own risk. Neither Menasha Ridge Press nor Robert Loewendick is liable for property loss or damage, personal injury, or death that result in any way from accessing or hiking the trails described in the following pages. Please be especially cautious when walking in potentially hazardous terrains with, for example, steep inclines or drop-offs. Do not attempt to explore terrain that may be beyond your abilities. Please read carefully the introduction to this book as well as further safety information from other sources. Familiarize yourself with current weather reports and maps of the area you plan to visit (in addition to the maps provided in this guidebook). Be cognizant of park regulations and always follow them. *Do not take chances.*

Contents

Dedication

To my wife, Linda, for sharing those days on the trails and for the years of dedication to our cherished friendship. And to my two children, Danielle and Rob, for exploring nature with me since their births.

Acknowledgments

I am the author that compiled the information and explored the trails, but I was blessed with several sources for recommendations, on-site direction, companionship, and editorial guidance. Without this support, the book would lack as a quality guide—I raise my hiking sticks and tip my hat to the following people in appreciation.

Walk into any of the nature centers near these trails and you'll be met with a smile and a quick offer to answer a question. The passion of those working at these centers is contagious. It was nearly as pleasing to listen to stories of the parks and preserves as it was to explore them myself. Other employees and volunteers I met along the way also provided a smile and were eager to share recommendations for trails and provided background information that made my visits pleasurable ones.

Fellow hikers I passed on the trail or chatted with at trailheads willingly shared hikes they favored and ones they would not care to do again—and explained why. It's always a pleasure to talk nature exploration with those who appreciate doing so by trail.

To my constant trail companion—my wife, Linda. Walking these trails was more enjoyable with you by my side. No matter the weather or adverse conditions, you presented a beautiful smile at the end of each hike. And to our grown children, Danielle and Rob, who explored with me and displayed two types of hiking's joys: thoroughly inspecting nature discoveries along the trail and the thrill of covering miles of a strenuous trail in good time. I loved every minute.

To Menasha Ridge Editors Susan Haynes, who guided my trail selection process, and Larry Bleiberg, for polishing my manuscript. And to Scott McGrew for understanding and assembling my GPS notes to create these detailed maps.

Preface

Fast-paced living has become the norm. Few of us take time to, as the adage goes, stop to smell the roses—or the wildflowers in this case. Getting out on a hiking trail and roaming a place set aside for its natural beauty help apply the brakes to a busy life. For many folks, the definition of hiking brings to mind cleated boots, backpacks, and body-length staffs whittled from tree saplings. The vision of a young man standing on a rock ledge overlooking a great valley completes the image. Hiking might seem unreachable for many of us, but in reality it's easy to detour from our busy lives by stepping onto a hiking trail. The only requirements: comfortable clothing for the season, a pair of running shoes, and a day pack to hold a bottle of water and a pocket-size first-aid kit. Oh, and one other thing—a hiking trail. But if you live in Columbus or one of the Capitol City's suburbs, you're in luck.

As a freelance outdoor writer, I frequently travel Ohio covering subjects that involve people of all ages. Numerous programs invite families and individuals to experience what the outdoors has to offer. Most folks are surprised to learn that so many opportunities are found so close to home. At a glance, central Ohio didn't appear to be a mecca for hiking. But after investigating a few trails over the years, I was pleasantly surprised with the possible hiking experiences, and searched out the best trails within a 90-minute drive of downtown Columbus—offering ample time for travel and to enjoy a day hike. As I continued hiking with a camera, GPS, and a voice recorder for note taking, central Ohio's hiking story kept growing into one I couldn't wait to write about.

Columbus has an impressive Metro Park system with all but one park within a few minutes' drive from Interstate 270. Diverse trail types—dirt, gravel, and paved—lead hikers through a variety of landscapes. The Battelle Darby Creek Metro Park covers more than 7,000 acres with two State and National Scenic Rivers flowing

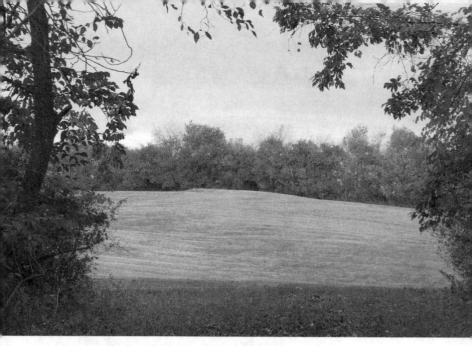

AN AMERICAN INDIAN MOUND WATCHES OVER THE TRAIL AT INFIRMARY MOUND PARK.

through the middle of it all. The diverse Chestnut Ridge Metro Park blankets a forested ridge and a wetland. The Sharon Woods Metro Park hosts a mixture of forests and meadows with vernal pools for springtime bird songs at dusk and a fishing lake for seniors and kids. Each park has its own atmosphere: some are more out of the city's shadow, while others border interstate highway fences. However, they all host trails that provide a pleasurable walk or invigorating ramble with interesting views and natural attractions.

Ohio's state parks, natural areas, and preserves are among the best in the country. The opportunities to add a night of camping to a day of hiking at a state park are many. Although each trail destination highlighted in this book can be tackled in one day, spending a couple of hours around a campfire sharing thoughts of the day's hike is icing on the cake. The state nature preserves are Ohio's quiet hiking gems. I hiked the Shallenberger Nature Preserve, north of Lancaster, twice while researching this book. Both times (weekends), I crossed paths with no one, either on the trail or in the parking lot.

Most of the Metro Park trails are well maintained with pavement or crushed limestone. Spur trails and secondary trails are either mowed paths through a meadow or packed-dirt, narrow trails near creeks and rivers. Nature preserves are just that—preservers of nature—so don't expect manicured trails. There is one noteworthy exception: a half-mile, concrete walkway up the center of Conkle's Hollow. State parks are also left in a natural state, and most are not maintained except for tree clearing. This adds to the wilderness flavor of several trails included in this book—an element appreciated by more aggressive hikers.

I have detailed these 31 hikes to assist in planning your next, or your first, hike in or around Columbus and central Ohio. As a treat, I've left a few pleasant surprises of each trail and trail location for you to discover on your own. Trekking up a hiking trail anticipating the view over the ridge or around the bend is a thrill. The diversity of this group of Five-Star trails keeps the hikes exciting from the first one to the last. There are more than 100 miles of trails introduced in this book, so snug up those shoelaces and get started.

Recommended Hikes

Best for Fall Color

Best for Geology

Best for Kids

Best for Picnics

Best for Scenery

Best for Seclusion

Best for Wildflowers

Best for Wildlife

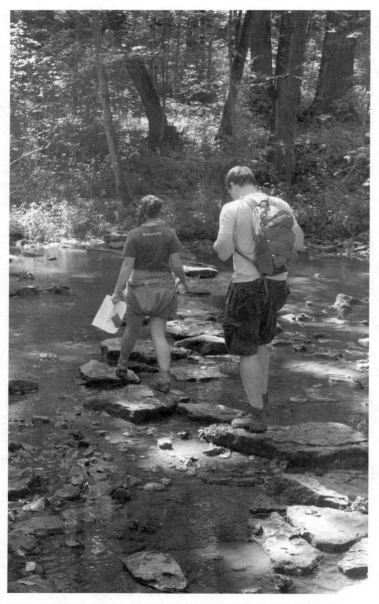

ROCK-HOPPING ACROSS A CREEK AT THE GLEN HELEN NATURE PRESERVE

Introduction

About This Book

Ohio's geographical diversity is as varied as any state. Narrow that view into central Ohio and the landscape and water bodies remain mixed. This book divides central Ohio into five regions: central, north, east, south, and west.

The central region (with the outer edge of Interstate 270 as its perimeter) includes mostly Metro Parks, each having its individual flair. On the west side of the region, Prairie Oaks Metro Park sits on both sides of the Big Darby Creek State and National Scenic River, with hiking trails flanking both sides of the waterway. To the east, along I-70, is Blacklick Woods Metro Park, which features a mixture of forest types, but no rivers. On the north side of the central region, Highbanks Metro Park's trails lead to a 100-foot cliff above another scenic river, the Olentangy. Although the central region was cleared of woodlands a couple of centuries ago, pockets of mature forests stand along with meadows and wetlands, creating a hiking delight.

The northern region stretches up to include Mohican and Malabar State Parks. Clear Fork Gorge and the Mohican River, another designated state Scenic River, offer trails to waterfalls and river views through a hemlock forest. Walking among the hemlocks and mossy boulders, you'll feel as if you're exploring a forest deep in the Appalachian Mountains.

The eastern region includes a blend of forests and fields, with small streams and a couple of rivers and their branches. Blackhand Gorge State Nature Preserve is well visited, but the trail there featured in this book runs the hills and hollows of a section that receives little traffic. You'll also find solitude hiking the Hebron Fish Hatchery in Licking County. Trails avoid the rearing ponds, instead exploring the hatchery's forest swamplands and ponds, several of which are hidden between woodlots and favored waterfowl haunts

1

during migration seasons. But watch your step, as the rarely seen massasauga rattlesnake inhabits the wet forest.

The Hocking Hills make up a majority of the southern region. This landscape has been cut and carved by glacial meltwaters, creating caves, gorges, and natural bridges. The king of the southeast hill country is Old Man's Cave. The gorge that includes the big cave and several additional rock formations is the most visited geological attraction in the state. To the west of the Hocking Hills, you'll find A. W. Marion State Park. The trail there encircles a picturesque, 145-acre lake with coves jetting into forested hollows. The lake and woods are surrounded by agricultural fields that were graded level by the last glacier.

Clifton Gorge State Nature Preserve and adjoining John Bryan State Park showcase another popular gorge with trails exploring rims and depths. This amazing geological landform and the Little Miami River that flows through it sit below the flat prairielands of the western region. Glen Helen Nature Preserve, a neighbor of John Bryan State Park, includes a yellow spring, soothing cascades, and various other works of nature for exploration. These parks and preserves are to the far west of Columbus but on the east side of Dayton.

Each hike was judged using a five-star rating system, detailed below. Although the selected hikes will not score a five in each category, overall each trip provides a five-star hiking experience.

How to Use This Guidebook

The following information walks you through this guidebook's organization to make it easy and convenient for planning great hikes.

Overview Map, Map Key, & Map Legend

The overview map on the inside front cover depicts the location of the primary trailhead for all 31 hikes. The numbers shown on the overview map pair with the map key on the facing page. Each hike's number remains with that hike throughout the book. Thus, if you spot an appealing hiking area on the overview map, you can flip through the book and find those hikes easily by their sequential numbers at the top of each profile page.

Trail Maps

In addition to the overview map on the inside cover, a detailed map of each hike's route appears with its profile. On each of these maps, symbols indicate the trailhead, the complete route, significant features, facilities, and topographic landmarks such as creeks, overlooks, and peaks. A legend identifying the map symbols used throughout the book appears on the inside back cover.

To produce the highly accurate maps in this book, I used a handheld GPS unit to gather data while hiking each route, and then sent that data to the publisher's expert cartographers. However, your GPS is not a substitute for sound, sensible navigation that takes into account the conditions that you observe while hiking.

Further, despite the high quality of the maps in this guidebook, the publisher and I strongly recommend that you always carry an additional map, such as the ones noted in each profile opener's "Maps" listing.

Elevation Profile

For trails with significant changes in elevation, the hike descriptions include this graphical element. Entries for fairly flat routes, such as a lake loop, do not display an elevation profile. Also, each entry's key information lists the elevation at the hike trailhead, as well as the route's highest point.

For hike descriptions that include an elevation profile, this diagram represents the rises and falls of the trail as viewed from the side, over the complete distance (in miles) of that trail. On the diagram's vertical axis, or height scale, the number of feet indicated between each tick mark lets you visualize the climb. To avoid making flat hikes look steep and steep hikes appear flat, varying height scales provide an accurate image of each hike's climbing challenge.

The Hike Profile

Each profile opens with the hike's star ratings, GPS trailhead coordinates, and other key at-a-glance information—from the trail's distance and configuration to contacts for local information. Each profile also includes a map (see "Trail Maps," above). The main text for each profile includes four sections: Overview, Route Details, Nearby Attractions, and Directions (for driving to the trailhead area).

Star Ratings

Five-Star Trails is the title of a Menasha Ridge Press guidebook series geared to specific cities across the United States, such as this one for Columbus. Following is the explanation for the rating system of one to five stars in each of the five categories for each hike.

FOR SCENERY:

★★★★★   Unique, picturesque panoramas

★★★★   Diverse vistas

★★★   Pleasant views

★★   Unchanging landscape

★   Not selected for scenery

FOR TRAIL CONDITION:

★★★★★   Consistently well maintained

★★★★   Stable, with no surprises

★★★   Average terrain to negotiate

★★   Inconsistent, with good and poor areas

★   Rocky, overgrown, or often muddy

FOR CHILDREN:

★★★★★   Babes in strollers are welcome

★★★★   Fun for anyone past the toddler stage

★★★   Good for young hikers with proven stamina

★★   Not enjoyable for children

★   Not advisable for children

FOR DIFFICULTY:

★★★★★   Grueling

★★★★   Strenuous

★ ★ ★   Moderate (won't beat you up—but you'll know you've been hiking)

★ ★   Easy with patches of moderate

★   Good for a relaxing stroll

FOR SOLITUDE:

★ ★ ★ ★ ★   Positively tranquil

★ ★ ★ ★   Spurts of isolation

★ ★ ★   Moderately secluded

★ ★   Crowded on weekends and holidays

★   Steady stream of individuals and/or groups

GPS TRAILHEAD COORDINATES

As noted in "Trail Maps," on page 3, I used a handheld GPS unit to obtain geographic data and sent the information to the cartographers at Menasha Ridge. In the opener for each hike profile, the coordinates—the intersection of the latitude (north) and longitude (west)—will orient you from the trailhead. In some cases, you can drive within viewing distance of a trailhead. Other hiking routes require a short walk to the trailhead from a parking area.

This guidebook uses the degree–decimal minute format for presenting GPS coordinates. The latitude–longitude grid system is likely quite familiar to you, but here is a refresher, pertinent to visualizing the GPS coordinates:

Imaginary lines of latitude—called parallels and approximately 69 miles apart from each other—run horizontally around the globe. The equator is established to be 0°, and each parallel is indicated by degrees from the equator: up to 90°N at the North Pole, and down to 90°S at the South Pole.

Imaginary lines of longitude—called meridians—run perpendicular to lines of latitude and are likewise indicated by degrees. Starting from 0° at the Prime Meridian in Greenwich, England, they continue to the east and west until they meet 180° later at the International Date Line in the Pacific Ocean. At the equator, longitude lines also are approximately 69 miles apart, but that distance narrows as the meridians converge toward the North and South Poles.

To convert GPS coordinates given in degrees, minutes, and seconds to degrees–decimal minutes, the seconds are divided by 60. For more on GPS technology, visit **usgs.gov.**

DISTANCE & CONFIGURATION

Distance indicates the length of the hike from start to finish, either round-trip or one-way depending on the trail configuration. If the hike description includes options to shorten or extend the hike, those distances will also be factored here. Configuration defines the type of route—for example, an out-and-back (which takes you in and out the same way), a figure eight, a loop, or a balloon.

HIKING TIME

A general rule of thumb for the hiking times noted in this guidebook is 1.5 miles per hour. That pace typically allows time for taking photos, for dawdling and admiring views, and for alternating stretches of hills and descents. When deciding whether or not to follow a particular trail in this guidebook, consider your own pace, the weather, your general physical condition, and your energy level that day.

HIGHLIGHTS

This section lists features that draw hikers to the trail: waterfalls, historic sites, and the like.

ELEVATION

In each hike's key information, you'll see the elevation (in feet) at the trailhead and another figure for the peak height on that route. For routes that involve significant ascents and descents, the hike profile also includes an elevation diagram (see page 3).

ACCESS

Fees or permits required to hike the trail are detailed here—and noted if there are none. Trail-access hours are also shown here.

MAPS

Resources for maps, in addition to those in this guidebook, are listed here. (As previously noted, the publisher and I recommend that you carry more than one map—and that you consult those maps before heading out on the trail in order to resolve any confusion or discrepancy.)

FACILITIES

This section alerts you to restrooms, phones, water, picnic tables, and other basics at or near the trailhead.

WHEELCHAIR ACCESS

Notes paved sections or other areas where one can safely use a wheelchair.

COMMENTS

Here you'll find assorted nuggets of information, such as whether or not dogs are allowed on the trails.

CONTACTS

Listed here are phone numbers and website addresses for checking trail conditions and gleaning other day-to-day information.

Overview, Route Details, Nearby Attractions, & Directions

These four elements provide the main text about the hike. "Overview" gives you a quick summary of what to expect on that trail; the "Route Details" guide you on the hike, start to finish; "Nearby Attractions" suggests appealing area sites, such as restaurants, museums, and other trails. "Directions" will get you to the trailhead from a well-known road or highway.

Weather

Hiking in central Ohio is a year-round activity, with extreme weather only on rare occasions. Winter hikes provide a needed escape from a season that can drag on for a few months. Visits to trails in the spring are welcomed with budding wildflowers, and blooming shows beckon hikers in summer and fall. The deciduous forests, which are common around every trail in this guide, provide a vibrant display of color as leaves change before dropping. However, autumn can be wet at times, creating a slippery situation with soaked leaves lying on the trail.

The following chart lists average temperatures and precipitation by month for the Columbus region. For each month, "Hi Temp" is the average daytime high; "Lo Temp" is the average nighttime low; and "Rain" is the average precipitation.

MONTH	HI TEMP	LO TEMP	RAIN or SNOW
January	36.2°F	20.3°F	2.53"
February	40.5°F	23.5°F	2.20"
March	51.7°F	32.2°F	2.89"
April	62.9°F	41.2°F	3.25"
May	73.3°F	51.8°F	3.88"
June	81.6°F	60.7°F	4.07"
July	85.3°F	64.9°F	4.61"
August	83.8°F	63.2°F	3.72"
September	77.1°F	55.9°F	2.92"
October	65.4°F	44.0°F	2.31"
November	52.4°F	34.9°F	3.19"
December	41.0°F	25.9°F	2.93"

Water

How much is enough? Well, one simple physiological fact should convince you to err on the side of excess when deciding how much water to pack: a hiker walking steadily in 90° heat needs approximately 10 quarts of fluid per day. That's 2.5 gallons. A good rule of thumb is to hydrate prior to your hike, carry (and drink) 6 ounces of water for every mile you plan to hike, and hydrate again after the hike. For most people, the pleasures of hiking make carrying water a relatively minor price to pay to remain safe and healthy. So pack more water than you anticipate needing even for short hikes.

If you're tempted to drink "found water," do so with extreme caution. Many ponds and lakes you'll encounter are fairly stagnant, and the water tastes terrible. Drinking such water presents inherent risks for thirsty trekkers. Giardia parasites contaminate many water sources and cause the dreaded intestinal giardiasis, which can last for weeks after onset. For more information, visit The Centers for Disease Control and Prevention website at **cdc.gov/parasites/giardia.**

In any case, effective treatment is essential before using any water source found along the trail. Boiling water for 2 to 3 minutes is always a safe measure for camping, but day hikers can consider iodine tablets, approved chemical mixes, filtration units rated for giardia, and UV filtration. Some of these methods (for example, filtration with an added carbon filter) remove bad tastes typical in stagnant water, while others add their own taste. As a precaution, carry a means of water purification to help in a pinch and if you realize you have underestimated your consumption needs.

Clothing

Weather, unexpected trail conditions, fatigue, extended hiking duration, and wrong turns can individually or collectively turn a great outing into a very uncomfortable one at best—and a life-threatening one at worst. Thus, proper attire plays a key role in staying comfortable and, sometimes, in staying alive. Here are some helpful guidelines:

Choose silk, wool, or synthetics for maximum comfort in all of your hiking attire—from hats to socks and in between. Cotton is fine if the weather remains dry and stable, but you won't be happy if that material gets wet.

Always wear a hat, or at least tuck one into your day pack or hitch it to your belt. Hats offer all-weather sun and wind protection as well as warmth if it turns cold.

Be ready to layer up or down as the day progresses and the mercury rises or falls. Today's outdoor wear makes layering easy,

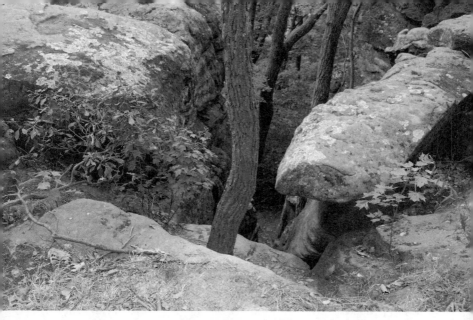

ENJOY THE CLIFF-TOP VIEW AT SHALLENBERGER STATE NATURE PRESERVE.

with such designs as jackets that convert to vests and zip-off or button-up legs.

Wear hiking boots or sturdy hiking sandals with toe protection. Flip-flopping along a paved urban greenway is one thing, but never hike a trail in open sandals or casual sneakers. Your bones and arches need support, and your skin needs protection.

Pair that footwear with good socks! If you prefer not to sheathe your feet when wearing hiking sandals, tuck the socks into your day pack; you may need them if the weather plummets or if you hit rocky turf and pebbles begin to irritate your feet. And, in an emergency, if you have lost your gloves, you can adapt the socks into mittens.

Don't leave rainwear behind, even if the day dawns clear and sunny. Tuck into your day pack, or tie around your waist, a jacket that is breathable and either water-resistant or waterproof. Investigate different choices at your local outdoors retailer. If you're a frequent hiker, ideally you'll have more than one rainwear weight, material, and style in your closet to protect you in all seasons in your regional climate and hiking microclimates.

Essential Gear

Today you can buy outdoor vests that have up to 20 pockets shaped and sized to carry everything from toothpicks to binoculars. Or, if you don't aspire to feel like a burro, you can neatly stow all of these items in your day pack or backpack. The following list showcases never-hike-without-them items—in alphabetical order, as all are important:

★ *Extra clothes:* raingear, a change of socks and shirt, and depending on the season, a warm hat and gloves.

★ *Extra food:* trail mix, granola bars, or other high-energy foods.

★ *Flashlight or headlamp* with extra bulb and batteries.

★ *Insect repellent.* For some areas and seasons, this is extremely vital.

★ *Maps and a high-quality compass.* Even if you know the terrain from previous hikes, don't leave home without these tools. And, as previously noted, bring maps in addition to those in this guidebook, and consult your maps prior to the hike. If you're GPS-savvy, bring that device, too, but don't rely on it as your sole navigational tool—battery life is limited, after all—and be sure to check its accuracy against that of your maps and compass.

★ *Pocketknife and/or multitool.*

★ *Sunscreen.* Check the expiration date on the tube or bottle.

★ *Water.* As emphasized more than once in this book, bring more than you think you'll drink. Depending on your destination, you may want to bring a container and iodine or a filter for purifying water in case you run out.

★ *Whistle.* It could become your best friend in an emergency.

★ *Windproof matches* and/or a lighter, as well as a fire starter.

First-Aid Kit

In addition to the items above, those below may appear overwhelming for a day hike. But any paramedic will tell you that the products listed here—again, in alphabetical order, because all are important—are just the basics. The reality of hiking is that you can be out for a week of backpacking and acquire only a mosquito bite. Or you can hike for an hour, slip, and suffer a bleeding abrasion or broken bone. Fortunately, these listed items will collapse into a very small space. You also may purchase convenient, prepackaged kits at your pharmacy or on the Internet.

★ Ace bandages or Spenco joint wraps

★ Adhesive bandages

★ Antibiotic ointment (Neosporin or the generic equivalent)

★ Athletic tape

★ Benadryl or the generic equivalent, diphenhydramine (in case of allergic reactions)

★ Blister kit (such as Moleskin or Spenco 2nd Skin)

★ Butterfly-closure bandages

★ Epinephrine in a prefilled syringe (typically by prescription only, and for people known to have severe allergic reactions to hiking mishaps such as bee stings)

★ Gauze (one roll and a half dozen 4-by-4-inch pads)

★ Hydrogen peroxide or iodine

★ Ibuprofen or acetaminophen

Note: Consider your intended terrain and the number of hikers in your party before you exclude any article listed above. A botanical garden stroll may not inspire you to carry a complete kit, but anything beyond that warrants precaution. When hiking alone, you should always be prepared for a medical need. And if you're a twosome or with a group, one or more people in your party should be equipped with first-aid material.

General Safety

The following tips may have the familiar ring of your mother's voice as you take note of them.

★ *Always let someone know where you'll be hiking and how long you expect to be gone.* It's a good idea to give that person a copy of your route, particularly if you're headed into any isolated area. Check in when you return.

★ *Always sign in and out of any trail registers provided.* Don't hesitate to comment on the trail condition if space is provided; that's your opportunity to alert others to any problems you encounter.

★ *Don't count on a cell phone for your safety.* Reception may be spotty or nonexistent on the trail, even on an urban walk—especially one embraced by towering trees or buildings.

★ *Always carry food and water, even for a short hike.* And bring more water than you think you'll need. (We can't emphasize this enough!)

★ *Ask questions.* Public-land employees are on hand to help. It's a lot easier to solicit advice before a problem occurs, and it will help you avoid a mishap away from civilization when it's too late to amend an error.

★ *Stay on designated trails.* Even on the most clearly marked trails, you usually reach a point where you have to stop and consider in which direction to head. If you become disoriented, don't panic. As soon as you think you may be off track, stop, assess your current direction, and then retrace your steps to the point where you went astray. Using a map, a compass, and this book, and keeping in mind what you've passed thus far, reorient yourself, and trust your judgment on which way to continue. If you become absolutely unsure of how to continue, return to your vehicle the way you came in. Should you become completely lost and have no idea how to find the trailhead, remaining in place along the trail and waiting for help is most often the best option for adults and always the best option for children.

★ *Always carry a whistle,* another precaution that we can't overemphasize. It may become a lifesaver if you get lost or hurt.

★ *Be especially careful when crossing streams.* Whether you're fording the stream or crossing on a log, make every step count. If you have any doubt about maintaining your balance on a log, ford the stream instead: use a trekking pole or stout stick for balance and face upstream as you cross. If a stream seems too deep to ford, turn back. Whatever is on the other side isn't worth risking your life for.

★ *Be careful at overlooks.* While these areas may provide spectacular views, they are potentially hazardous. Stay back from the edge of outcrops, and make absolutely sure of your footing; a misstep can mean a nasty and possibly fatal fall.

★ *Standing dead trees and storm-damaged living trees pose a significant hazard to hikers.* These trees may have loose or broken limbs that could fall at any time. While walking beneath trees, and when choosing a spot to rest or enjoy your snack, look up!

★ *Know the symptoms of subnormal body temperature, or hypothermia.* Shivering and forgetfulness are the two most common indicators of this stealthy killer. Hypothermia can occur at any elevation, even in the summer, especially when the hiker is wearing lightweight cotton clothing. If symptoms develop, get to shelter, hot liquids, and dry clothes ASAP.

★ *Likewise, know the symptoms of heat exhaustion, or hyperthermia.* Lightheadedness and loss of energy of the first two indicators. If you feel these symptoms, find some shade, drink your water, remove as many layers of clothing as practical, and stay put until you cool down. Marching through heat exhaustion leads to heatstroke—which can be fatal. If you should be sweating and you're not, that's the signature warning sign. Your hike is over at that point—heatstroke is a life-threatening condition that can cause seizures, convulsions, and eventually death. If you or a companion reaches that point, do whatever you can to cool down, and seek medical attention immediately.

★ *Most importantly, take along your brain.* A cool, calculating mind is the single-most important asset on the trail. It allows you to think before you act.

★ *In summary:* Plan ahead. Watch your step. Avoid accidents before they happen. Enjoy a rewarding and relaxing hike.

Watchwords for Flora & Fauna

Hikers should remain aware of the following concerns regarding plant life and wildlife, described in alphabetical order.

Black Bears

Though sightings of black bears are very rare, and attacks more so, the sight or approach of a bear can give anyone a start. If you encounter a bear while hiking, remain calm and avoid running in any direction. Make loud noises to scare off the bear and back away slowly. In primitive and remote areas, assume bears are present; in more-developed sites, check on the current bear situation prior to hiking. Most encounters are food-related, as bears have an exceptional sense of smell and not particularly discriminating tastes. While this is of greater concern to backpackers and campers, on a day hike, you may plan a lunchtime picnic or will munch on a power bar or other snack from time to time. So remain aware and alert.

Black Flies

Though certainly a maddening annoyance, a black fly will at worst cause an itchy welt. They are most active from mid-May into June, during the day, and especially before thunderstorms, as well as during the morning and evening. Insect repellent has some effect, though the only way to keep out of their swarming midst is to keep moving.

Mosquitoes

Ward off these pests with insect repellent and/or repellent-impregnated clothing. In some areas, mosquitoes are known to carry the West Nile virus, so take extra care to avoid their bites.

Poison Ivy & Sumac

Recognizing and avoiding poison ivy and sumac are the most effective ways to prevent the painful, itchy rashes associated with these plants. Poison ivy occurs as a vine or groundcover, three leaflets to a leaf; and poison sumac flourishes in swampland, each leaf having 7–13 leaflets. Urushiol, the oil in the sap of these plants, is responsible for the rash. Within 14 hours of exposure, raised lines and/or blisters will appear on the affected area, accompanied by a terrible itch. Refrain from scratching, because bacteria under your fingernails can cause an infection. Wash and dry the affected area thoroughly, applying a calamine lotion to help dry out the rash. If itching or blistering is severe, seek medical attention. To keep from spreading the misery to someone else, wash not only any exposed parts of your body but also any oil-contaminated clothes, hiking gear, and pets. Long pants and a long-sleeved shirt may offer the best protection.

Snakes

Rattlesnakes, cottonmouths, copperheads, and corals are among the most common venomous snakes in the United States, and their hibernation season is typically October–April. But despite their fearsome reputation, rattlesnakes like to bask in the sun and won't bite unless threatened.

In the region described in this book, you'll possibly encounter copperheads and rattlesnakes. However, the snakes you most likely will see while hiking will be nonvenomous species and subspecies. The best rule is to leave all snakes alone, give them a wide berth as you hike past, and be sure any hiking companions (including dogs) do the same.

When hiking, stick to well-used trails, and wear over-the-ankle boots and loose-fitting long pants. Do not step or put your hands beyond your range of detailed visibility, and avoid wandering around in the dark. Step onto logs and rocks, never over them, and be especially careful when climbing rocks. Always avoid walking through dense brush or willow thickets.

Ticks

These arachnids are often found on brush and tall grass, where they seem to be waiting to hitch a ride on warm-blooded passersby. Adult ticks are most active April–May and again October–November. The black-legged (deer) tick is the primary carrier of Lyme disease.

A few precautions: Wear light-colored clothing, which will make it easy to spot ticks before they migrate to your skin. After hiking, inspect your hair, the back of your neck, your armpits, and your socks. During your posthike shower, take a moment to do a more complete body check. To remove a tick that is already embedded, use tweezers made just for this purpose. Treat the bite with disinfectant solution.

Hunting

A number of rules, regulations, and licenses govern the various hunting types and related seasons. Though no problems generally arise, hikers may wish to forgo their trips during the big-game seasons, when the woods suddenly seem filled with orange and camouflage.

Regulations

Each state generally has a unique set of regulations that applies to the use of its parks and other public lands. Below you will find the rules that are most important to know when visiting these areas.

★ No pets permitted (except assistance animals) in nature preserves.

★ No collection of any plant, animal, or other substance permitted in nature preserves.

★ No swimming or wading permitted in nature preserves.

★ Visitors are required to stay on trails in nature preserves.

Trail Etiquette

Always treat trails, wildlife, and fellow hikers with respect. Here are some reminders.

★ *Plan ahead in order to be self-sufficient at all times.* For example, carry necessary supplies for changes in weather or other conditions. A well-planned trip brings satisfaction to you and to others.

★ *Hike on open trails only.*

★ *In seasons or construction areas where road or trail closures may be a possibility,* use the website addresses or phone numbers shown in the "Contacts" line for each of this guidebook's hikes to check conditions prior to heading out for your hike. And do not attempt to circumvent such closures.

★ *Avoid trespassing on private land, and obtain all permits and authorization as required.* Also, leave gates as you found them or as directed by signage.

★ *Be courteous to other hikers, bikers, equestrians, and others you encounter on the trails.*

★ *Never spook wild animals or pets.* An unannounced approach, a sudden movement, or a loud noise startles most critters, and a surprised animal can be dangerous to you, to others, and to itself. Give animals plenty of space.

★ *Observe the* YIELD *signs around the region's trailheads and backcountry.* Typically they advise hikers to yield to horses, and bikers to yield to both horses and hikers. Observing common courtesy on hills, hikers and bikers yield to any uphill traffic. When encountering mounted riders or horse packers, hikers can courteously step off the trail, on the downhill side if possible. So that horses can see and hear you, calmly greet their riders before they reach you, and do not dart behind trees. Also resist the urge to pet horses unless you're invited to do so.

★ *Stay on the existing trail and do not blaze any new trails.*

★ *Be sure to pack out what you pack in, leaving only your footprints.* No one likes to see the trash someone else has left behind.

Tips on Enjoying Hiking in Columbus

Storms gain momentum gliding across western Ohio, so when they arrive in Columbus, they pack a punch. Call park or preserve offices to confirm trails are open. The clay soils under some of the trails don't absorb rainwater quickly, so expect to tread through mud or puddles even a couple of days after a rain. During summer, vegetation can grow onto the trail; wear long pants to avoid scratches and insect bites.

The Metro Parks see the most visitors because of their proximity to suburbs. Early mornings provide the best chance for a hike with few others on the trail. The paved Metro Park trails are shared with cyclists, so listen for an approaching rider shouting a passing signal. The unpaved trails attract cross-country runners, and the same goes for these athletes, shouting warnings of passing on the left or right.

State nature preserves receive the least traffic, which is fantastic for solitude-seekers, but vandalism can occur at parking areas that have little to no security surveillance. Leave valuables at home—do not store them in your vehicle. In an emergency, you should be able to get cell phone service on nearly all of the trails in this book, except for the Hocking Hills region.

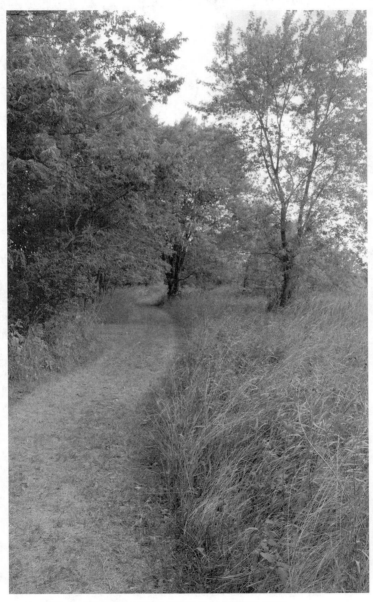

A MOWED TRAIL FOLLOWS A MEADOW EDGE AT STAGE'S POND
STATE NATURE PRESERVE.

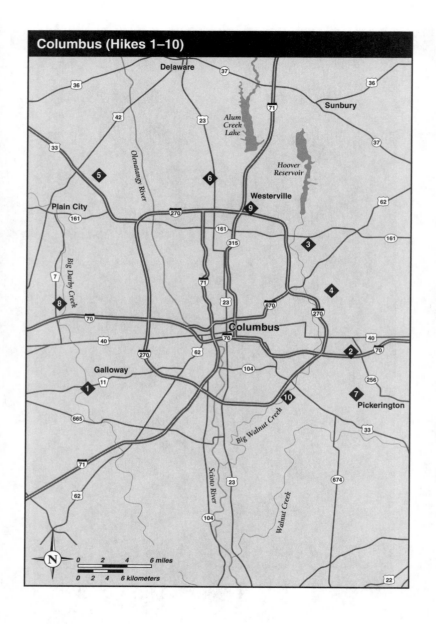

Columbus (Hikes 1–10)

Central

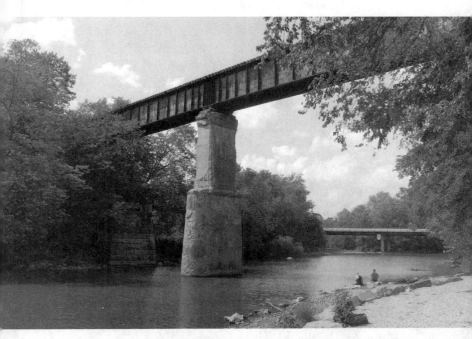

TAKE A BREAK AND ENJOY A REFRESHING FOOT SOAKING IN BIG DARBY CREEK.

Battelle Darby Creek Metro Park

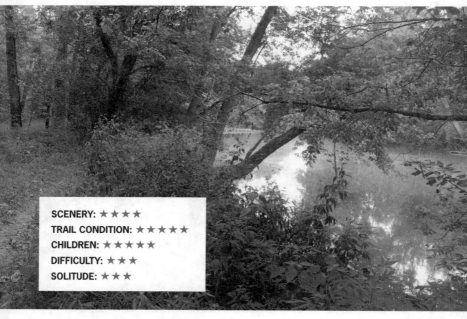

SCENERY: ★ ★ ★ ★
TRAIL CONDITION: ★ ★ ★ ★ ★
CHILDREN: ★ ★ ★ ★ ★
DIFFICULTY: ★ ★ ★
SOLITUDE: ★ ★ ★

A CREEKSIDE TRAIL FOLLOWS DARBY CREEK.

GPS TRAILHEAD COORDINATES: N39° 53.490' W83° 12.787'

DISTANCE & CONFIGURATION: 3.9-mile figure eight

HIKING TIME: About 3 hours

HIGHLIGHTS: Woodlands, American Indian mound, creeks

ELEVATION: 855' at trailhead to 928' at highest point

ACCESS: April–September: daily, 6:30 a.m.–10 p.m.; October–March: daily, 6:30 a.m.–8 p.m.

MAPS: At bulletin boards, **tinyurl.com/battelledarby**

FACILITIES: Restrooms, drinking water, picnic areas, playground, Natural Play Area

WHEELCHAIR ACCESS: Only on the Darby Creek Greenway Trail

COMMENTS: The Natural Play Area allows children to experience hands-on nature activities. Pets and bicycles prohibited on nature trails.

CONTACTS: 1775 Darby Creek Drive, Galloway, OH 43119; 614-891-0700; **tinyurl.com/battelledarby**

Overview

Battelle Darby Creek is the largest park in the Metro Park system. The Big Darby and Little Darby Creeks, both designated State and National Scenic Rivers, run through its center. The Ancient Trail travels along the Big Darby where American Indians once maintained a village. The Terrace Trail explores a forest standing 100 feet above the fertile creek bottom. The blend of prairies, woodlands, and waterways creates an oasis for wildlife—and wildlife observers. The 7,060-acre park offers lots to see and do, and a hike is a great way to get started.

Route Details

Adventures abound year-round at Battelle Darby Creek Metro Park. You'll find picnic areas for free use, lodge rentals, fishing ponds, creek access, sledding, cross-country skiing, skating, canoeing and kayaking, a Natural Play Area for the kids, a public hunting area, and, of course, hiking. The park's landscape and waterways are as diverse as the activities they support. The trails detailed here feature two types of environments—creek bottomland and deciduous forest.

The Indian Ridge Picnic Area lies in the center of the park, but it may be the park's least-used picnic area. From the north side, near a restroom, the Terrace Trail starts into the woods. The trail is wide, topped with crushed limestone, and well graded. The winding climb up the hillside is not abrupt, but a gradual incline that still gets the blood flowing. A trailside interpretive sign provides facts about wildlife species that inhabit the area, while a nearby bench offers a good resting spot. As the hill levels out, you'll cross the park road on which you entered.

The forest opens up with less understory and larger-trunked hardwoods as the trail curves back toward the west. This stretch of deciduous forest provides the perfect setting for practicing tree identification. Consider bringing along an Eastern forest guidebook and see just how many different species you can recognize. At 1.1 miles the trail passes a piece of modern history, which many visitors

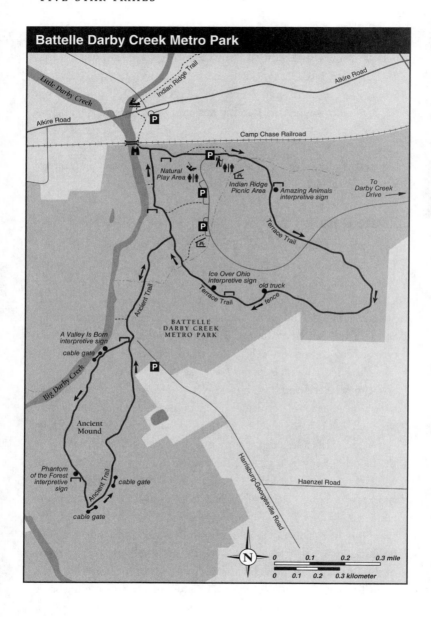

Battelle Darby Creek Metro Park

Little Darby Creek

Indian Ridge Trail

Alkire Road

Alkire Road

Camp Chase Railroad

P

P

Natural
Play Area

Indian Ridge
Picnic Area

Amazing Animals
interpretive sign

To
Darby Creek
Drive

P

Terrace Trail

Ancient Trail

Ice Over Ohio
interpretive sign

old truck

Terrace Trail

fence

BATTELLE
DARBY CREEK
METRO PARK

A Valley Is Born
interpretive sign

cable gate

Big Darby Creek

P

Ancient
Mound

Phantom
of the Forest
interpretive
sign

Ancient Trail

cable gate

Harrisburg-Georgesville Road

Haenzel Road

cable gate

N

| 0 | 0.1 | 0.2 | 0.3 mile |

| 0 | 0.1 | 0.2 | 0.3 kilometer |

will miss unless it's a season with no vegetation. Then it sticks out like an old truck—because that's what it is, or what's left of it. To the right of the trail you'll see a rusty red object sitting in the woods. A slim path makes its way to what's left of the 1950s Chevrolet.

The trail continues through oaks and maples and down an appealing ravine with rocks from hand-size to those measuring a few feet in diameter scattered about the seasonal creek bed. A bench and interpretive sign sit on the edge of this ravine. The sign reveals how today's landscape was carved out during the last glacial period, which also produced the peculiar looking stones. Leave the forest briefly and cross an opening dotted with wildflowers and shrubs. Then you'll enter a younger woodland, and at 1.5 miles reach the Ancient Trail intersection on the left.

Follow the Ancient Trail along Big Darby Creek and its creek-bottom habitat. Wildflowers and riparian plants grow under the sporadic tree canopy shading most of the creek bank. Not only is the Big Darby a scenic river to view and paddle, but also the river's underwater environment is just as appealing. The creek, which seems as wide as a river, supports threatened and endangered fish and mussels. Both the

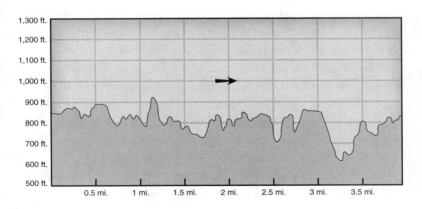

Big Darby's and Little Darby's mussels have been considered by some aquatic experts as the most diverse collection in North America.

A rise in the land takes the hike to the north corner of a meadow of approximately 50 acres. Also at this point is the dead end of Harrisburg-Georgesville Road. Signage here informs visitors arriving in vehicles that parking is allowed and points out the trail directions. The trail appears to be a dirt farm road with stands of trees on both sides.

Positioned just above the creek and along the meadow's edge, at 2.2 miles, is the Ancient Mound. A comprehensive interpretive sign inspires many to gaze across the meadow and imagine what the long-gone American Indian village would have actually looked like. Nearly 1,000 years ago, what is now a meadow of wildflowers was then a field growing the "three sisters": maize, beans, and squash. Now follow the trail on the mowed path south, then east, then north to return to the point where the road dead-ends, and enjoy the shaded walk to the Terrace Trail.

On the Terrace Trail, 3.6 miles into the hike, an intersecting dirt footpath leads down to the creek. The pathway to the Big Darby Creek is an extension of the 8-acre Natural Play Area that spreads out through the trees and shrubs to the right. Kids and accompanying adults are encouraged to take a hands-on approach as they explore the forest and creek. About 400 feet straight ahead, the Terrace Trail is met on the left by the Indian Ridge Trail. Turn left and walk about 100 feet around the bend to find a scenic vista of the Big Darby and Little Darby confluence. An iron train trestle crosses overhead, and creekside rocks, the perfect size to sit on with feet dangling in the water, line the gravel beach between creek and trail. Two interpretive signs stand here too, revealing the history of the railroad passing by and sharing white-tailed deer facts. Turn around and return to the Terrace Trail. Hike east 0.1 mile to an opening through the brush on the right, which leads to the Indian Ridge Picnic Area and your ride.

Nearby Attractions

With more than 7,000 acres of park, you shouldn't have any trouble finding something interesting nearby. At the north end of the park, walk the Darby Creek Greenway Trail, starting at the Cedar Ridge entrance and parking area near the park office. Travel north on the wide gravel multiuse trail for about 1 mile to reach the fields that hold several bison—yes, buffalo. To the south of the park center, just south of Interstate 71, on the outskirts of Springlawn off OH 3, you'll find a small fishing lake and a couple of miles of hiking trails circling the lake and passing through a woodlot and prairie.

Directions

From I-270 take Exit 7 and travel west on US 40 for 5.1 miles to Darby Creek Drive. Turn left and continue south 4.1 miles to the Indian Ridge entrance on the right.

Blacklick Woods Metro Park

SCENERY: ★ ★ ★
TRAIL CONDITION: ★ ★ ★ ★ ★
CHILDREN: ★ ★ ★ ★ ★
DIFFICULTY: ★
SOLITUDE: ★ ★

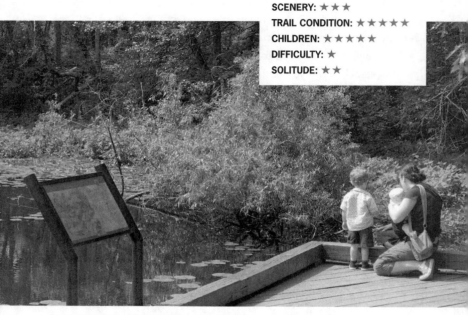

A MOTHER AND HER CHILDREN OBSERVE THE ABUNDANT POND LIFE.

GPS TRAILHEAD COORDINATES: N39° 56.021' W82° 48.372'

DISTANCE & CONFIGURATION: 2.3-mile loop

HIKING TIME: About 1.5 hours

HIGHLIGHTS: Hardwood swamp, boardwalk, pond, birding

ELEVATION: 749' at trailhead; 650' to 906' overall

ACCESS: January–March and October–December: daily, 6:30 a.m.–8 p.m.;
April–September: daily, 6:30 a.m.–10 p.m.

MAPS: At bulletin boards in parking areas, nature center, and **tinyurl.com/blacklick**

FACILITIES: Restrooms, drinking water, nature center

WHEELCHAIR ACCESS: On Beech and Buttonbush Trails

COMMENTS: Off-trail activity is prohibited in the nature preserve;
pets not permitted on trails.

CONTACTS: 6975 E. Livingston Avenue, Reynoldsburg, OH 43068; 614-891-0700;
tinyurl.com/blacklick

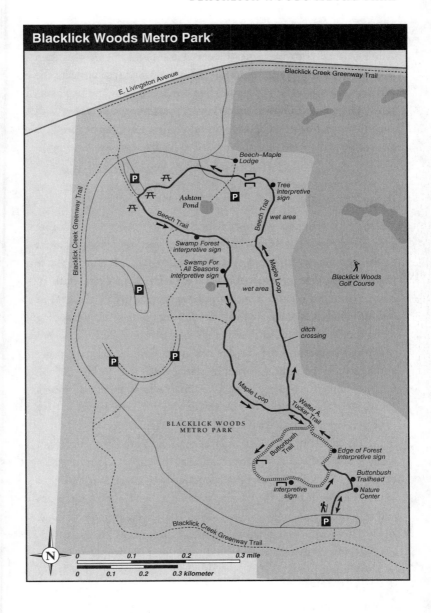

Blacklick Woods Metro Park

E. Livingston Avenue

Blacklick Creek Greenway Trail

Blacklick Creek Greenway Trail

Beech–Maple Lodge

Tree interpretive sign

Ashton Pond

Beech Trail

Beech Trail

wet area

Swamp Forest interpretive sign

Swamp For All Seasons interpretive sign

wet area

Maple Loop

Blacklick Woods Golf Course

ditch crossing

Maple Loop

Walter A. Tucker Trail

BLACKLICK WOODS METRO PARK

Buttonbush Trail

Edge of Forest interpretive sign

Buttonbush Trailhead

Nature Center

interpretive sign

Blacklick Creek Greenway Trail

0   0.1   0.2   0.3 mile

0   0.1   0.2   0.3 kilometer

N

Overview

A brick paved path welcomes hikers at the parking area and then leads to the nature center and the trailhead. This hike connects the Buttonbush, Walter A. Tucker, Maple Loop, and Beech Trails to make one round route. The first section runs along the edge of a woodland swamp and a forest, while the second section explores deeper into the hardwood forest. The third section encircles a woodland pond and passes through a picnic area and playgrounds.

Route Details

When this metro park was established in 1948, it was the first of its kind in central Ohio. As concern grew about the loss of natural areas as the capital city expanded into the countryside, the now 643-acre park soon became a treasured natural area. Even with Interstate 70 buzzing along the park's southern border, and with a tight grid of residential dwellings on the west side and shopping centers standing along the east side, the park remains a quiet place to disappear from the madness that modern-day life can create. Hardwood trees cover almost half of the park, and our hike plan investigates the heart of the forest. A forest of hickory, beech, and maple trees creates a birder's paradise. In the spring, listen for the hooting of barred owls as they maintain several nests, especially along the Maple Loop.

We begin our hike at the southern parking area, which you can easily find by following signage starting at the entrance on the park's north side. Look for a brick paved walkway with a trail map sign that enters the woods from the parking area's northern edge. A restroom and water fountain are a few yards to the left of the paved entryway. The walkway leads to the nature center, which features a covered deck area and interactive displays geared to all ages. Buttonbush Trail, a crushed limestone path, is more than 10 feet wide, well groomed, and leads into the woods just north of the nature center. Soon a boardwalk comes in from the left—you will return from that direction. To the right is a 3-foot round boulder with an attached plaque marking the dedication of the Blacklick Woods' Walter A. Tucker Preserve as a Registered Natural Landmark. Tucker was the Metro Park system's first executive director.

When the Buttonbush Trail begins to cross fingers of a woodland swamp, sections of boardwalk replace the stone path. At 0.4 mile the 0.1-mile Walter A. Tucker Connector Trail sneaks off to the right and joins the Maple Loop trail. Take the connector and enjoy the view of the surrounding hardwoods and get a whiff of the woodsy aroma. This second section remains in the forest. A golf course borders the right side of the trail but doesn't impose on the hike's natural setting. On most days, a refreshing breeze comes off the golf course and filters into the woods and over the trail. From the point the connector trail meets the Maple Loop, the path continues on a fairly straight stretch for 0.4 mile through a forest of maple and beech trees then T's into the Beech Trail, where you'll take a right.

While hiking the Metro Parks, you'll often find small interpretive signs. On the Beech Trail, signs include tree species identification and forest habitat notes. At the 1-mile mark, a path to the right leads to the Beech-Maple Lodge. At the same location, a trail turns left and ends at a small parking area in the woods. A short trail leads away from that parking area and arrives at Ashton Pond and an observation deck complete with chairs. The pond is a must-see addition to this hike—be sure your camera has a fresh set of batteries. The multitude of fish-slurping bugs from the surface and turtles coming out for a peek-and-eat session are entertaining.

Back on the Beech Trail, the path becomes paved after leaving the pond's parking area. At 0.1 mile from the parking area, the trail breaks into an open picnic and playground area, dotted with shade trees and parking. This picnic area gets pretty busy most days, even during the week. But don't worry; the trail reenters the woods after a brief run through the picnic area, and returns to nature. The Maple Loop joins the Beech Trail at the second point at the 1.4-mile mark—go this way. The southbound portion of the Maple Loop should be hiked with attentive ears. This stretch of forest has hosted an owl's nest for several years. During my research hike there, I heard and saw a mature barred owl perched high in a tree. Sit on the bench located a few hundred feet from the last trail intersection and listen for the owls or the dozens of other bird species that inhabit the preserve.

At the 1.5-mile mark, a spur trail takes off to the right (west) and ends at a cluster of three reservable picnic areas. Continue on the Maple Loop for another 0.25 mile to return to the Walter A. Tucker Connector Trail, which you passed earlier. Follow the connector trail back to the Buttonbush Trail and take a right. This last curve of the hike includes a few stints of boardwalks leapfrogged with stone path stretches (the last 0.2 mile is boardwalk). Take a right at the Registered Natural Landmark rock to return to the nature center.

Nearby Attractions

Pickerington Ponds Metro Park is 3 miles south. Its hiking trail is level and easygoing. The ponds are popular with various waterfowl during migrations in fall and spring.

Directions

From I-270, take the East Main Street/Reynoldsburg exit. Go east on Main Street (US 40) to Brice Road and turn right. Follow Brice Road to Livingston Avenue and turn left. The park entrance is about 1.2 miles on the right.

Blendon Woods Metro Park

SCENERY: ★ ★ ★
TRAIL CONDITION: ★ ★ ★ ★ ★
CHILDREN: ★ ★ ★ ★ ★
DIFFICULTY: ★ ★
SOLITUDE: ★ ★

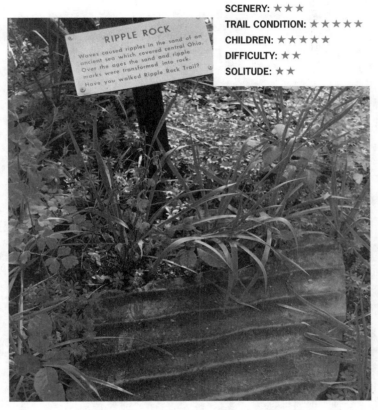

RIPPLE ROCK

Waves caused ripples in the sand of an ancient sea which covered central Ohio. Over the ages the sand and ripple marks were transformed into rock. Have you walked Ripple Rock Trail?

THIS RIPPLE ROCK IS EVIDENCE THAT THE LAND WAS ONCE COVERED BY AN ANCIENT SEA.

GPS TRAILHEAD COORDINATES: N40° 04.284' W82° 52.411'

DISTANCE & CONFIGURATION: 2.4-mile balloon with spur

HIKING TIME: About 1 hour

HIGHLIGHTS: Woodland creek, waterfowl-watching, deciduous forest

ELEVATION: 922' at trailhead; 661' to 994' overall

ACCESS: January–March and October–December: daily, 6:30 a.m.–8 p.m.; April–September: daily, 6:30 a.m.–10 p.m.

MAPS: At bulletin boards in parking areas, nature center, and **tinyurl.com/blendonwoods**

Blendon Woods Metro Park

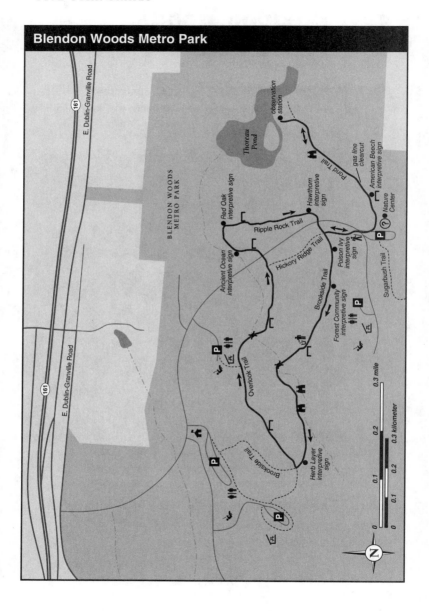

FACILITIES: Restrooms, drinking water, nature center, ranger station, sports courts

WHEELCHAIR ACCESS: Yes, on Pond Trail

COMMENTS: Off-trail activity is prohibited in Walden Waterfowl Refuge.

CONTACTS: 4265 E. Dublin-Granville Road, Westerville, OH 43081; 614-891-0700; tinyurl.com/blendonwoods

Overview

A walk in the woods drops down a ridge to stroll by a woodland creek that includes two crossings on footbridges. A short stint on a connector trail brings you back by your vehicle, but before leaving, a level, paved trail cuts through a woodland and ends at a waterfowl refuge with two wildlife observation blinds. A nature center filled with flora and fauna demands a visit before wrapping up a day in this pretty park. This hike combines the Brookside, Overlook, Ripple Rock, Pond, and Hickory Ridge Trails.

Route Details

Expect to spend more time at this park than the hour allotted for the hike. Driving in, it soon becomes evident that these 653 acres are a refuge from the urban jungle surrounding them. Half of the park is covered with forest, consisting primarily of oaks, hickories, and maples—which all light up with colors in the fall. A deep gully cuts through the center of the park, and two of the trails you will be hiking explore this ravine floor as well as the ridges on both sides. Bring your binoculars during the spring birding season.

From the main entrance on the park's north border, drive past the ranger station and the Shadblow Reservable Area, both on the right, and follow the signs to the nature center. Park next to the center and begin the hike there. If the nature center is closed, check the bulletin board in the center of the parking area for any trail alerts or postings of wildlife sightings. Walk to the park road to the parking area entrance, and look for the Hickory Ridge Trail trailhead across the road. Follow the 10-foot-wide crushed limestone–packed trail for 0.1 mile to the intersection with the Brookside Trail and go left (west) on the Brookside Trail. As with all of the Columbus Metro Parks, interpretive signs along the trails identify tree and plant species. The next stretch of trail guides you through a pleasant forest environment. Along the way, one of those interpretive signs (most are rectangle-shaped aluminum, about 6 by 12 inches) on the right provides information on Blendon Woods' forest community. You'll learn, for example, that the park hosts more than 40 native trees.

The trail holds true to its name as it follows a woodland brook for about 0.1 mile after crossing a 40-foot bridge at the 0.4-mile point. Pause at the trail's edge to check out the brook's aquatic life. A set of binoculars is not only a great tool for watching songbirds darting from limb to limb, but also works well for spying on minnows and crawdads snatching up larvae downstream. At 0.7 mile the Brookside Trail intersects the Overlook Trail—go right and head to the northeast on the Overlook Trail. The trail goes uphill, still surrounded by forest. About 0.3 mile from the last intersection, a small path joins the Overlook Trail from the left. This path connects the Shadlow Reservable Area to the main route and is intended only for picnickers' access.

The Overlook Trail crosses the creek on a wooden footbridge, and then soon delivers you back up on the initial ridge, where you'll continue east. A pleasant view of the forested ravine continues for a few hundred feet before it gives way to a young mix of hardwood forest. At 1.2 miles, the Hickory Ridge Trail meets the Overlook Trail from the right. If you want to turn back, take the Hickory Ridge Trail to your vehicle. If not, proceed to cross the park road using the painted crosswalk. It leads to the Ripple Rock Trail, which rounds a forested hillside with a parade of small interpretive signs paralleling the path. Pieces of flat stone topped with rows of ridges are found in the adjacent creek. The ripples on the unique rocks were formed by waves of an ancient sea that once covered Ohio.

Ripple Rock Trail crosses the park road and soon joins Brookside Trail and Hickory Ridge Trail to the left. Follow the Hickory Ridge Trail south to the point where you began the hike at the parking area. You could call it a day, but since your muscles are warm and ready, why not steer yourself to the nature center and the start of the paved Pond Trail? This 0.3-mile jaunt leads to your choice of two observation shelters (with spotting scopes) situated on the edge of Thoreau Lake, in the middle of Walden Waterfowl Refuge. A variety of ducks, including the hooded merganser, pause at the lake during migration seasons. More than 220 bird species have been spotted at the park. If the nature center is open when you return to the parking area, duck inside (no pun intended) to see what else has been found in the park.

Nearby Attractions

Two miles to the southwest, the Easton area offers dozens of restaurants, entertainment, and shopping—including a couple of major sporting goods stores. Another 5 miles to the northwest, sister metro park Sharon Woods offers 3 miles of nature trails.

Directions

From Interstate 270, Exit 30 B, take OH 161 east onto E. Dublin-Granville Road for 1.6 miles. Take the Little Turtle Way exit and turn right, then take another right at the light onto Cherry Bottom Road, traveling west. Park entrance is 0.5 mile on the left.

4 # Gahanna Woods:
City Park and State Nature Preserve

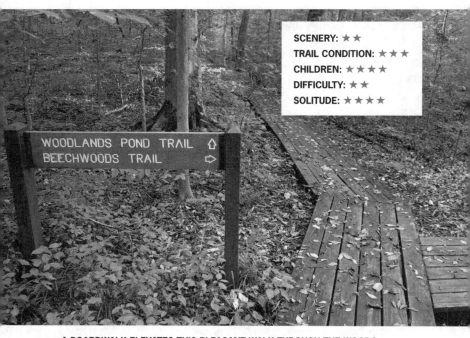

SCENERY: ★ ★
TRAIL CONDITION: ★ ★ ★
CHILDREN: ★ ★ ★ ★
DIFFICULTY: ★ ★
SOLITUDE: ★ ★ ★ ★

WOODLANDS POND TRAIL ⬆
BEECHWOODS TRAIL ⮕

A BOARDWALK ELEVATES THIS PLEASANT WALK THROUGH THE WOODS.

GPS TRAILHEAD COORDINATES: N40° 00.705' W82° 50.095'

DISTANCE & CONFIGURATION: 1.9-mile loop

HIKING TIME: About 1.5 hours

HIGHLIGHTS: Woodlands, wildlife

ELEVATION: 887' at trailhead, with no significant rise

ACCESS: Daily, sunrise–sunset; no permits required

MAPS: Posted on bulletin boards

FACILITIES: None

WHEELCHAIR ACCESS: No

COMMENTS: Bicycles are permitted on paved path through city park section.

CONTACTS: 1501 Taylor Station Road, Gahanna, OH 43230; 614-342-4250;
tinyurl.com/gahanna

Overview

The partnering of a city park with a neighboring state nature preserve creates a quick but nature-filled getaway without leaving the city. Walk a paved maintenance road to escape the parking area, and 100 yards later a few grassy trail options appear. Travel a figure eight through a woodlot tucked behind a subdivision where tall pines provide a peaceful setting and a pleasing aroma. Pop back out at the parking lot and then glide into a more secluded portion of the hike. The Gahanna Woods State Nature Preserve hosts the southern half of this trek; it's fairly quiet except for the jets from Port Columbus International Airport 2 miles away. Nearly the entire hike is immersed in woodlands, and more than half traverses swamp habitat.

Route Details

Green spaces are a priority for many cities across the United States. The Columbus suburb of Gahanna supports that quest for preserving natural places while providing access to residents and visitors alike. Two governing bodies, the City of Gahanna and Ohio's Division of Natural Areas and Preserves, manage two adjoining properties as one. The nearly 100 acres of natural bounty are squeezed by a subdivision on two sides and an industrial park on another. Even so, the nearly 2-mile hike through these woods is a pleasant one with long spells of silence except for whistling songbirds—oh, and an airliner a couple of times each hour.

The parking lot serves as basecamp for the hike, as you will return there when you finish the city park section and on your way to the state nature preserve. This makes a great setup if young children are on your adventure team and need a drink and snack mid-trip. From the paved parking lot, follow the paved park road north toward the water tower rising above the trees. Two small spur trails veer off to the right, swinging through a mowed meadow sporting bird boxes on stakes. The park road continues north to the water tower. This same roadway is a thoroughfare for bicyclists pedaling through the

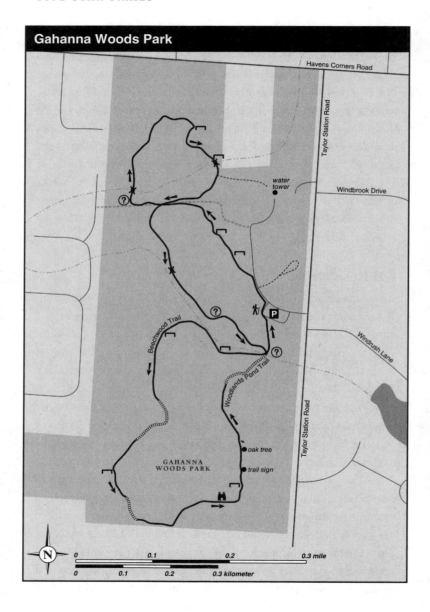

Gahanna Woods Park

park from the neighborhood to the west to Taylor Station Road on the east side of the property. Bikes are not allowed on any other park trails or in the nature preserve.

Across the park road from the two small spur trails is an 8-foot-wide mowed path leading into a short forest of shrubs and saplings. Follow that trail but go slowly, as there is more wildlife in this city park than you might think; try not to spook it away before you can observe it. Various species of flowering shrubs, wildflowers, and weeds border the trail and provide food for the wild critters hanging out there. Don't expect to see deeper into the more mature forest in the center of the park from this stretch of trail, unless hiking during winter. Multiple benches placed trailside throughout the park encourage visitors to slow down and unwind.

At 0.3 mile the mowed trail meets a gravel lane. This path is an extension of the paved lane leading to the water tower and connecting to the neighborhood to the west, and is the bicycle route mentioned earlier. Follow the gravel lane (passing a couple of trail intersections) to the west until you reach the bulletin board at the bike entrance. Follow the mowed path north from the bulletin board, cross the small footbridge, and enter a pine forest surrounded by deciduous trees. The scent of the tall conifers more than makes up for the road noise coming from the north, out of sight. Continue looping around and meet the gravel lane again at the same point where you came up from the south. Again, follow the gravel lane to the west, but this time turn left (south) at the trail before reaching the bulletin board—creating a figure-eight pattern before returning to the parking area.

The trail surface is cushioned by mulch at several points, which helps keep it mud-free. The vegetation stands closer to the trail in this section, narrowing the path, but it's not leg-rubbing close. Watch for meadow mushrooms growing trailside during late summer and early fall. Nearly year-round you'll hear insects communicating their messages and amusing hikers with their songs. Enter the lawn area of the city park and walk south of the parking area (or take that break at the car) to the bulletin board standing next to the trail leading into the woods—the entrance to Gahanna Woods State Nature Preserve.

Take a peek at the bulletin board for any current warnings from nature preserve management. Cross the footbridge over a small stream and turn right past the large brown preserve sign to the split in the trail. A sign identifies the two trails that explore the preserve—follow the Woodlands Pond Trail. It will turn north and come close to the city park trail you were just on, but once deep into the woods, it turns slowly south. A bench and somewhat open area in the understory allow for watching warblers and thrushes flittering about. Several mature beech trees stand guard over the swamp forest that stays moist year-round except during extremely dry weather. Between here and the western park boundary you'll encounter four shallow marsh ponds, which brim with life during the spring, when peepers and insects nearly drown out the sound of jets overhead. The Woodlands Pond Trail leads off to the east at 1.3 miles, and the Beechwood Trail continues south—follow the Beechwood Trail.

At 1.5 miles the Beechwood Trail turns east, passing through the heart of a beech-dominated forest. At this point, it's as secluded as it gets at Gahanna Woods. During my hike there, I paused to make a note, and a white-tailed doe and her fawn stood from a bedding position to observe me—only 15 yards between us. The fawn was jittery, but its mother stood her ground and watched me walk away; she never ran. The wildlife of Gahanna Woods have clearly adapted to the presence of people, cars, and wandering pets. Take advantage of the benches to sit and blend into the woods for a few minutes and see what emerges to observe you or simply to go about its routine. At 1.7 miles the Woodlands Pond Trail joins from the west. The understory gets thicker and the trail narrows for the last 200 feet before returning to the nature preserve entrance.

Nearby Attractions

Creekside Park and Plaza is 3 miles west of Gahanna Woods Park on OH 317. This 5-acre park on Big Walnut Creek offers biking, boating (rentals available), and creek wading for a dose of natural fun. For man-made amusement, its shopping, dining, events, and live entertainment fill the bill.

Directions

From I-270 Exit 37, follow OH 317 (South Hamilton Road) north 0.8 mile to Havens Corners Road and turn right (east). Travel 1.7 miles to Taylor Station Road and turn right. The park entrance is on the right in 0.4 mile.

Glacier Ridge Metro Park

SCENERY: ★ ★ ★
TRAIL CONDITION: ★ ★ ★ ★ ★
CHILDREN: ★ ★ ★ ★ ★
DIFFICULTY: ★
SOLITUDE: ★ ★

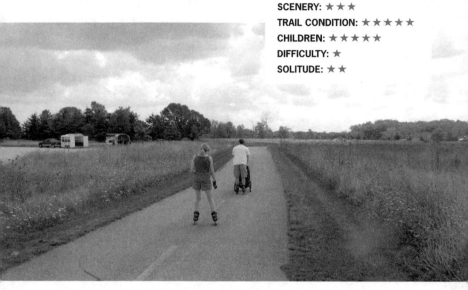

THE PAVED TRAIL ATTRACTS WHEELED ADVENTURERS AS WELL AS HIKERS.

GPS TRAILHEAD COORDINATES: N40° 09.272' W83° 11.760'

DISTANCE & CONFIGURATION: 2.8-mile loop

HIKING TIME: About 2 hours

HIGHLIGHTS: Meadows, woodlots, outdoor learning center

ELEVATION: 1,006' at trailhead, with no significant rise

ACCESS: Year-round, daily, 6:30 a.m.–sunset

MAPS: At bulletin boards and **tinyurl.com/glacierridgepark**

FACILITIES: Restrooms, drinking water, picnic areas, playground, wind and solar learning center

WHEELCHAIR ACCESS: Yes

COMMENTS: The disc golf course covers 20 acres, and parts of the course cross the Marsh Hawk Trail near the Bridle Trail Staging Area.

CONTACTS: 9801 Hyland Croy Road, Plain City, OH 43064; 614-891-0700; **tinyurl.com/glacierridgepark**

Overview

Walk the prairie covering a rise in the flat landscape that was created by a receding glacier 15,000 years ago. Urban sprawl has worked its way up from Columbus, but is held at bay by the Glacier Ridge Metro Park. The Marsh Hawk Trail takes hikers in a big circle, but it's not a boring stroll in the park. Vernal pools, wetlands, woodscapes, grasslands, and a wind and solar learning center are the life of this hiking party.

Route Details

The moraine (an accumulation of earthen materials) left by the glacier is hardly noticeable as a ridge at Glacier Ridge Metro Park. Instead, it's seen in a slightly sloping landscape devoid of geological features normally associated with a ridge site. There are no gorge cuts or caves to probe, but hikers will find more than 1,000 acres of natural landscape worthy of exploring. No ropes or spiked shoes needed at this park—a comfortable pair of sneakers will suffice to handle this level, relaxing stroll.

The center of the park's main section is a windmill producing electricity, and spread around its base is a circuitry of solar panels and controls. This is the Wind and Solar Learning Center—an interactive demo outdoor classroom. Both systems are described in detail with interpretive signs. The electricity produced here is fed into the local electric cooperative's grid. The working display is a must-see and demands at least 20 minutes for exploration.

You can begin the hike from the parking lot at the wind and solar center by walking the paved path near the bulletin board to the southwest. Or take the park road loop and park at the lot ahead near a restroom and water fountain. Either way, a paved access trail to the Marsh Hawk Trail leaves the center circle to the west and intersects the main loop of the trail. Turn right (north) at the T, and keep an eye and ear out for bicyclists or in-line skaters coming up from behind. This paved trail is also popular with runners, but we hikers provide a good showing too.

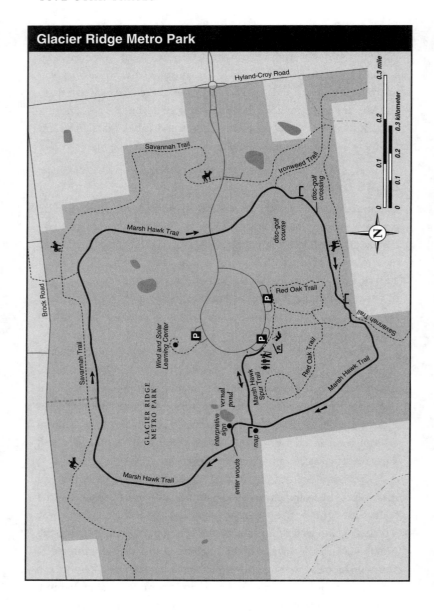

Glacier Ridge Metro Park

Hyland-Croy Road

Savannah Trail

Ironweed Trail

disc-golf crossing

disc-golf course

Marsh Hawk Trail

Brock Road

Red Oak Trail

P

P

P

Wind and Solar Learning Center

Savannah Trail

Savannah Trail

Red Oak Trail

Red Oak Trail

Marsh Hawk Trail

Marsh Hawk Spur Trail

GLACIER RIDGE METRO PARK

interpretive sign

vernal pond

map

enter woods

Marsh Hawk Trail

0.3 mile

0.3 kilometer

0.1   0.2

0   0.1   0.2

0

N

Just before the trail enters a woodlot, a recently created vernal pond sits in the meadow to the right. It will take 20 years or so, but the young trees surrounding it eventually will create a swampy forest to entertain the next generation. The north half of this hike cuts through the open prairie. Wildflowers galore paint this country throughout the growing seasons. The hairy sunflower's yellow petals spread and glow in August, and the tall ironweed's purple blooms attract butterflies in September and even into October.

The trail reaches a northeast bend, then turns south. If you can arrange to arrive at this point as the sun sets, you'll be positioned for a gorgeous sky show of color if the weather is right. It's a miniature version of the Big Sky effect found out West. Cross the main park road that you arrived on, and on the right you'll find another access path for the Marsh Hawk Trail (this one leads to the center of our hike and the parking areas). Back on the main loop, the meadow to the right has fewer wildflowers but more flying saucers. An 18-hole disc-golf course tests the saucer-flinging skills of anyone attempting the challenging but fun course—for free. To the left, the Ironweed Trail comes from the Honda Wetland Education Center at the most southern point of the park. A dozen yards south of that junction is a bench. It seems like a pleasant resting spot near the trail's halfway mark, but watch for flying discs, as a target basket (a disc golf "hole") stands just a few yards to the east.

The trail passes through the disc golf course and, turning west, enters a block of mature forest. Soon, the gravel Red Oak Trail passes by on the right as it makes its loop through the woods and back to the parking areas. Bird-watching is the activity of choice through this forest passage, especially in the morning. At 2.1 miles, the Marsh Hawk Trail leaves the woods and enters a meadow dotted with young shrubs and saplings. Another paved access trail comes in on the right from the parking area. Bear left and swing around the brushy meadow and north to another forest block. As you pass through the woods, the Red Oak Trail again passes close on the right, and the bridle trail flanks the Marsh Hawk Trail on the left. Leave the forest and immediately on the right you'll find the access trail you started on. If you didn't stop on the way in, take a moment now at the field edge and read the interpretive sign outlining the reforestation plans that will continue to build this park into something special.

Nearby Attractions

Two miles south of the park's main section is an extension of Glacier Ridge Metro Park. The Honda Wetland Education Area is a restored 250-acre area. A 22-foot observation tower provides a bird's-eye view of the ecosystem, while an education center and boardwalk offer up-close exploration. From the Honda Wetland Education Area, the Ironweed Trail leads north 2.8 miles to the park section surrounding the Wind and Solar Learning Center. You can access Honda Wetland Education Area by vehicle from Hyland-Croy Road, across from Tullymore Drive.

Directions

From I-270 Exit 17, follow US 33 west for 2.5 miles to the Post Road exit. Turn right (east) and then immediately left on Hyland-Croy Road. Travel north for 3.2 miles to a roundabout and circle around to head west into the park entrance.

Highbanks Metro Park

SCENERY: ★ ★ ★
TRAIL CONDITION: ★ ★ ★ ★ ★
CHILDREN: ★ ★ ★ ★
DIFFICULTY: ★ ★ ★
SOLITUDE: ★ ★

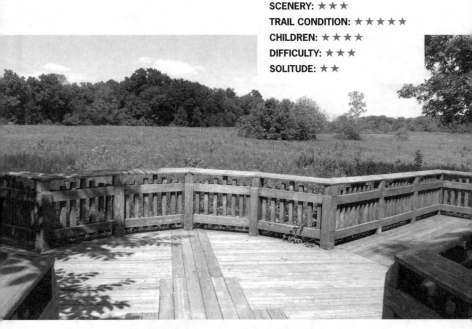

AN OBSERVATION DECK GIVES HIKERS A FRONT-ROW SEAT FOR A WILDLIFE SHOW IN THE MEADOW.

GPS TRAILHEAD COORDINATES: N40° 09.086' W83° 01.452'

DISTANCE & CONFIGURATION: 4.8-mile figure eight

HIKING TIME: About 3 hours

HIGHLIGHTS: Steep ravines, earthworks

ELEVATION: 917' at trailhead, with no significant rise

ACCESS: October–March: daily, 6:30 a.m.–8 p.m.; April–September: daily, 6:30 a.m.–10 p.m.

MAPS: At bulletin boards, nature center, **tinyurl.com/highbankspark**

FACILITIES: Nature center, picnic areas, restrooms, drinking water

WHEELCHAIR ACCESS: No, but yes on other trails at this park

COMMENTS: Off-trail activities are prohibited in the Edward F. Hutchins Nature Preserve and on the land surrounding the wetland and wetland viewing deck.

CONTACTS: 9466 Columbus Pike, Lewis Center, OH 43035; 614-891-0700; **tinyurl.com/highbankspark**

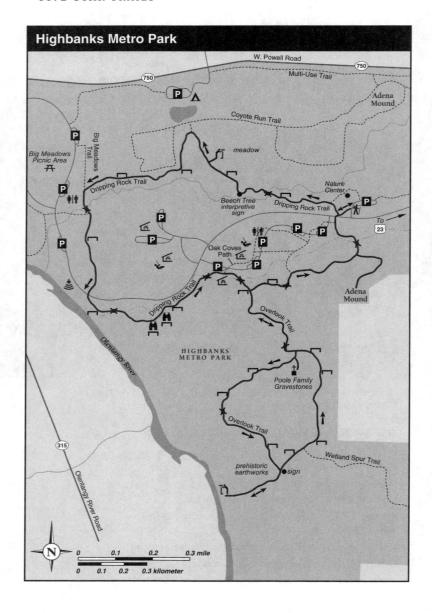

Highbanks Metro Park

W. Powell Road

750

Multi-Use Trail

750

Adena Mound

Coyote Run Trail

Big Meadows Trail

Big Meadows Picnic Area

Dripping Rock Trail

meadow

Beech Tree interpretive sign

Nature Center

Dripping Rock Trail

To 23

Oak Coves Path

Dripping Rock Trail

Adena Mound

Overlook Trail

Olentangy River

HIGHBANKS METRO PARK

Poole Family Gravestones

Overlook Trail

315

Olentangy River Road

prehistoric earthworks

sign

Wetland Spur Trail

N

0   0.1   0.2   0.3 mile

0   0.1   0.2   0.3 kilometer

Overview

Before the hike, tour the comprehensive nature center to learn about the landscape. Tread through a forest to an observation deck at a meadow's edge. Continue your walk through the woods and cross a few creeks on footbridges before arriving at the Overlook Trail. Pause at a small collection of gravestones and learn what life was like here two centuries ago. Pass through a break in prehistoric earthworks and reach the deck overlooking the Olentangy State Scenic River. Rejoin the Dripping Rock Trail and visit an Adena Indian mound before returning to the nature center.

Route Details

The Olentangy State Scenic River flows across a bed of limestone at the western edge of Highbanks Metro Park. The soft shale was cut by glacial meltwater, leaving behind a series of ravines. The landscape is now covered with forest and a few meadow openings. A visit to the nature center will reveal fossils found along the creeks that still are cutting into the ravine walls, promising that more fossils will be exposed in the future. While walking the trails here, be sure to pause

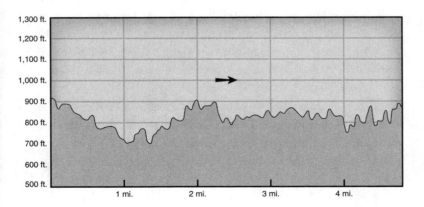

on the footbridges for a good look at the open layers of shale rock by the side of the stream.

From the nature center, walk west to find the Dripping Rock Trail crossing the park road. Stay on the north side of the road and follow the path north into the forest. The healthy, clean hardwood forest shades the trail with a canopy of oaks and maples. At 0.3 mile you'll encounter the first of many creek footbridges. An observation deck at 0.5 mile offers the first meadow view, and an interpretive sign explains the rutting ritual of the white-tailed deer. During the end of October and the first couple of weeks in November, bucks deviate from their normal reclusive habits and search for a receptive doe for breeding. Normally, it's easiest to observe deer early or late in the day, but during the breeding season bucks can be seen running all day. Keep a camera at the ready.

The trail narrows a few feet from the previous 12-foot-wide path, but remains well maintained throughout the park. Just 0.2 mile from the meadow observation deck, a short spur trail on the right leads to the Coyote Run Trail, which is designated as a pet trail and a cross-country skiing course. Drift over a crest and work along the upper edge of a ravine lined with rail fence. Nearing the bottom of the descent, a spur trail on the right leads to a parking area at the sledding hill and crosses the Big Meadows Trail near the park road. A couple hundred more feet along the Dripping Rock Trail, the Big Meadows Trail comes in from the right. The Big Meadows Trail crosses the park road to access the Scenic River Trail—a 0.6-mile walk along the river.

The Dripping Rock Trail continues south and slides under the park road, which passes overhead. Although there might be an occasional hum from passing vehicles, the sounds of a woodland filled with songbirds and insects predominate. The trail curves up to a ridgetop, passing three benches on the way. These benches, which sit along a stretch of trail on a quiet slope away from the picnic areas, offer a spot to view the shallow ravines and ridges just a few yards away. At 1.8 miles, the trail leaves the woods and passes through a parking area at the Oak Coves Picnic Area—a popular spot in the center of the park. The Oak Coves Path joins the Dripping Rock Trail at that point and follows the park road toward the nature center.

Stay on the Dripping Rock Trail to bear right and reenter the forest. After about 100 yards, the Overlook Trail comes in from the right. Follow the Overlook Trail to a meadow and walk the woods' edge for another 100 yards, with zigzagging butterflies and songbirds keeping you company out in the open. Back under forest cover and across a bridge, you'll find a split in the trail to the right, basically the western half of a looping trail—either way, the only way out is back to this point. A few steps down the western side of the Overlook Trail is a short spur to the Poole Family Gravestones. The markers are real, but the cemetery is not. The re-created burial ground honors some of the area's earliest settlers, who arrived in the early 1800s. The actual gravesites are unknown, but the stones were discovered near the park.

The Overlook Trail enters the Edward F. Hutchins State Nature Preserve at 2.5 miles. All state nature preserve rules apply here: visitors must stay on trails; no pets allowed; no collection of any plant, animal, or any other substance permitted; and no wading or swimming in creeks. A bridge that crosses a steep and deep ravine provides a great view of the process of erosion. The ravine is so deep that the trees growing near the ravine bottom don't reach the bridge deck—hikers walk over the treetops. An interpretive sign at the bridge explains how the ravine was created and what plant species grow in the ravine's cool environment.

At 2.8 miles the western half of the Overlook Trail meets the eastern half. Signposts suggest making a right turn to view the prehistoric earthworks and then standing on the overlook deck 100 feet above the Olentangy River—you must see both. The Cole Earthwork consists of three elongated mounds built by American Indians during the late Woodland period. Interestingly, a portion of the clay used to create the mounds is not found in the park and must have been carried here from farther downriver. Hike 0.2 mile from the earthwork to reach the deck above the river. You'll get the best water views in autumn. Viewed from above, the colorful blanket of leaves on the riverbanks makes a memorable photo.

Leave the deck and earthwork and follow the Overlook Trail, staying to the right at the east-west trail junction. At 3.2 miles the Wetland Spur Trail heads to the right and arrives at an observation deck at the wetland. Stay on the Overlook Trail and return to the Dripping Rock Trail. Travel east on Dripping Rock, bypassing a spur to the left at 4 miles that leads to the Oak Coves Path, and arriving at the spur trail on the right at 4.2 miles that leads to the small Adena Mound. From the head of the Adena Mound spur trail, trek north 0.2 mile to the nature center.

Nearby Attractions

The Columbus Zoo and Aquarium is 4 miles west of Highbanks Metro Park. Alum Creek State Park is 4 miles to the northeast and offers nearly 300 campsites, camper cabins, a 7-mile multipurpose trail, and 3,387 acres of lake to explore, fish, or swim. The park includes the largest inland swimming beach in Ohio's state park system—3,000 feet long.

Directions

From I-270 Exit 23, travel north on US 23 for 3 miles to the park entrance on the left.

7 # Pickerington Ponds
Metro Park

SCENERY: ★ ★ ★
TRAIL CONDITION: ★ ★ ★ ★ ★
CHILDREN: ★ ★ ★ ★
DIFFICULTY: ★ ★
SOLITUDE: ★ ★ ★ ★

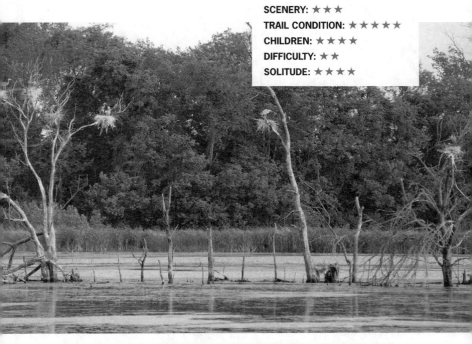

NESTING HERONS ARE JUST ONE OF THE NUMEROUS WILDLIFE SPECIES THAT LIVE IN AND AROUND THE PONDS.

GPS TRAILHEAD COORDINATES: N39° 53.087′ W82° 47.917′

DISTANCE & CONFIGURATION: 3.2-mile out-and-back

HIKING TIME: About 2.5 hours

HIGHLIGHTS: Heron rookery and waterfowl observatory, wide meadows

ELEVATION: 757′ at trailhead, with no significant rise

ACCESS: Daily, 6:30 a.m.–sunset

MAPS: At bulletin boards in parking areas and **tinyurl.com/pickerington**

FACILITIES: Restrooms, drinking water, nature center

WHEELCHAIR ACCESS: No

COMMENTS: Off-trail activity is prohibited in the nature preserve.

CONTACTS: 7680 Wright Road, Canal Winchester, OH 43110; 614-891-0700;
tinyurl.com/pickerington

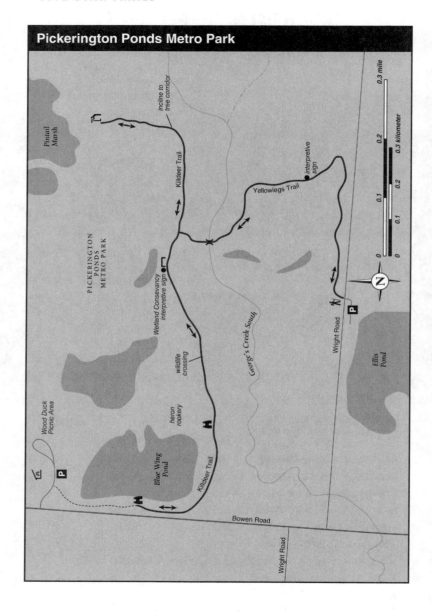

Pickerington Ponds Metro Park

Overview

The park is separated into four sections by two intersecting county roads. This hike follows the Yellow Legs and Killdeer Trails to explore the more remote section of the four. You'll pass through an open meadow that encircles a wetland, then cross a bridge over a stream. More meadow hiking leads to the out-of-the-way Pintail Marsh and its observation deck. Finally, you'll swing back around through the second meadow and view three ponds, one of which hosts an impressive heron rookery.

Route Details

Birds, birds, and more birds are what you will find while hiking this park. The blend of marshlands, ponds, and wooded lots create the right recipe for luring migrating waterfowl and shorebirds. Birders consider Pickerington one of the elite watching areas in central Ohio: it was designated an Ohio Important Birding Area by Audubon Ohio. The star attraction is the heron rookery, which you will find all lined up in the Blue Wing Pond and visit on this hike. You can easily observe the rookery from a parking area on the pond's north shore.

The parking lot on the south side of Wright Road overlooks Ellis Pond to the south. Park there, but turn around and cross Wright Road in the crosswalk, near the park office, to reach the Yellowlegs Trailhead. On the park trail map, the Yellowlegs path follows the eastern edge of what looks to be a pond, but it's actually a wetland with the trail passing 100 yards east of the wetland edge, before turning north and then west. During summer, the trail's jaunt through a field will let hikers witness swallows catching insects by the beakful. For springtime hikes, go slow and use binoculars as you traverse the field to catch a glimpse of a fox hunting mice.

At 0.6 mile the trail crosses a reconstructed road bridge. The tractor-wide crushed limestone path serves as an access road for park maintenance folks, and it also provides hikers a view of the sky to watch the abundance of birdlife jetting over from pond to pond, and meadow to wood line. Take a closer look at the stream with those birding binoculars hanging around your neck. Search for snapping turtles, crawfish, and brown water snakes maneuvering along the stream bank. One hundred feet beyond the bridge, the Yellowlegs Trail meets the Killdeer Trail—turn right here and travel east.

The trail immediately passes through a tree row and into a field surrounded by narrow, long woodlots and, to the south, a tree-lined creek bank. Seeming like a large courtyard inside a live tree fort, the field provides a protected location for hunting meals. Glance at the ground occasionally and you will likely find dried scat left by one of the wildlife species hunting here. Could you identify a scat sample? No? Pick up a pocket guide on the subject and educate yourself. At the east end of this yard (slightly larger than a football field), the trail turns north and into tree cover. The deciduous tree corridor serves as a living hallway with an observation deck and bench at the end—1 mile from the Yellowlegs Trailhead.

During spring and fall migration periods, dozens of waterfowl species can be seen here. It's best to hike at Pickerington Ponds when you have an extra hour, which will assure ample time to scope the ponds with binoculars and update your birding journal. From this observation deck, I watched two osprey dive-bomb Pintail Marsh, to the north, and snatch up unsuspecting prey in the seasonal ponds to the west. The impressive aerial show lasted for more than 30 minutes; I would have missed it if I was hurried.

Return to the intersection of Yellowlegs and Killdeer Trails, but this time continue on Killdeer. This trail flows straight for nearly 0.5 mile before turning north to the Blue Wing Pond parking area and observation point. On the way to that turnaround point, you will have a few opportunities to observe additional waterfowl shows in the sky to the north. The trail toward Blue Wing Pond is mowed a couple of yards wide on each side. Keep your eyes open for wildlife darting across the path. After spending some time at the parking area overlooking Blue Wing Pond and its rookery, along with flocks of geese, ducks, and, of course, blue herons, return to the Yellowlegs

Trail and continue to retrace your steps back across the bridge, through the first meadow, and to your ride home.

Nearby Attractions

The village of Pickerington, 2 miles east of the Metro Park, has a variety of restaurants and retail stores. Blacklick Woods Metro Park (3 miles north of the park) offers the Walter A. Tucker Nature Preserve, where you can explore a woodland swamp on hiking trails and boardwalks.

Directions

From I-270, take US 33 south for 4.7 miles to the OH 674/Gender Road exit. Travel north 2 miles to Wright Road and turn right. Go east 1 mile to Bowen Road and turn right; take the next left and drive 0.4 mile to the parking area on the right. The Yellowlegs Trailhead is across the road from the parking area entrance.

8

Prairie Oaks Metro Park

SCENERY: ★ ★ ★
TRAIL CONDITION: ★ ★ ★ ★ ★
CHILDREN: ★ ★ ★ ★ ★
DIFFICULTY: ★ ★ ★
SOLITUDE: ★ ★ ★

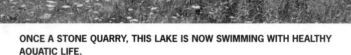

ONCE A STONE QUARRY, THIS LAKE IS NOW SWIMMING WITH HEALTHY AQUATIC LIFE.

GPS TRAILHEAD COORDINATES: N39° 59.634' W83° 15.524'

DISTANCE & CONFIGURATION: 5.3-mile figure eight

HIKING TIME: About 3 hours

HIGHLIGHTS: Lakes, creek, meadow

ELEVATION: 899' at trailhead, with no significant rise

ACCESS: Daily, 6:30 a.m.–sunset

MAPS: At bulletin boards and **tinyurl.com/prairieoaks**

FACILITIES: Restrooms, drinking water, picnic areas, playground, natural play area

WHEELCHAIR ACCESS: No

COMMENTS: Equestrians are allowed on the south stretch of the Lake View Trail and the midsection of the Coneflower Trail.

CONTACTS: 3225 Plain City–Georgesville Road, West Jefferson, OH 43162; 614-891-0700; **tinyurl.com/prairieoaks**

Overview

The 2,203-acre park sits on what was some of Ohio's greatest prairie lands before early settlers arrived and began to change the landscape. Today, the rich soils of the Darby Creek Watershed again host native prairie plants thanks to park managers and staff. A maze of trails covers the park with plenty of options for a variety of nature interaction. Two meadows of wildflowers and tall grasses make plenty of wildlife sightings likely. You'll slide by three deep-blue quarry lakes, where fishing is permitted, and climb the Sycamore Trail along the Big Darby Creek bottomlands. This hike includes the Darby Creek, Lake View, Alder, Sycamore, and Coneflower Trails.

Route Details

As Interstate 70 rolls west 10 miles out of Columbus, this pleasant and quiet Metro Park provides an escape from fast-paced city life. Big Darby Creek, designated as a State and National Scenic River, flows through the heart of the park, and a bridge crossing gives an overview of the special creek-bottom environment. The natural diversity is about as varied as any in the Columbus Metro Park collection. If you are short on time, take a quick workout hike. But if you have a day for a soak-it-all-in paced hike, Prairie Oaks Metro Park is the perfect setting, with creekside, grasslands, lakeside, and woodland hiking.

Arriving from Plain City–Georgesville Road on the park's west side, park at the Whispering Oaks Picnic Area, home to a first-class shelter for grilling and gathering. A dozen yards east you'll find the Darby Creek Greenway Trail running north and south. This wide gravel trail (more like a well-graded and maintained roadway) snakes through a meadow that demands a wildflower identification book. At 0.4 mile the trail reaches a steel-frame, wood-decked bridge over Big Darby Creek. Cross it and take an immediate left turn, staying on the Greenway Trail. Lake View and Alder Trails meet at the east end of the bridge as well—you will return to this point later in the hike, twice actually.

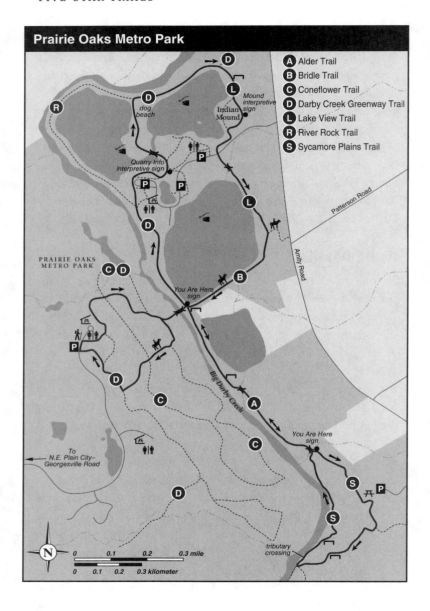

Prairie Oaks Metro Park

- **A** Alder Trail
- **B** Bridle Trail
- **C** Coneflower Trail
- **D** Darby Creek Greenway Trail
- **L** Lake View Trail
- **R** River Rock Trail
- **S** Sycamore Plains Trail

Patterson Road

Amity Road

dog beach

Mound interpretive sign

Indian Mound

Quarry Info interpretive sign

PRAIRIE OAKS METRO PARK

You Are Here sign

Big Darby Creek

You Are Here sign

To N.E. Plain City– Georgesville Road

tributary crossing

N

0   0.1   0.2   0.3 mile

0   0.1   0.2   0.3 kilometer

As the Greenway Trail continues north, the lake on the right is the first of three bodies of water you'll see on this hike. All are fishable, and two allow non-motorized boating. The lake water to the right is a deep-blue color with a brushy shoreline. This park section is the most visited, with picnic areas within a short walk of all three lakes. As you pass by, keep an eye out for the wetland-loving spotted turtle floating at the lake's edge—it's a small turtle with yellow spots painted over a black shell. The Darby Bend Lakes vehicle entrance is located on Amity Road.

The breeze off the lake rustles the leaves of aspen trees trailside, creating a treat for the senses. At 0.9 mile the River Rock Trail comes in on the left. This path loops around the lake coming into view on the left and later rejoins the Greenway Trail. Two gravel pathways that connect the picnic shelter areas to the hiking trails and lakes intersect the trail from the right. On the mowed lawn area on the east side of the Greenway Trail, you'll find a large chunk of limestone and an interpretive sign. It explains how the area transformed from quarry to a beautiful park.

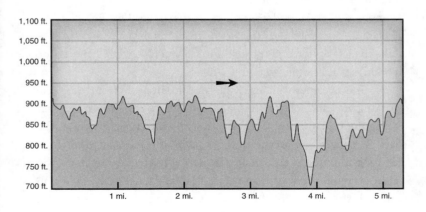

Cross a low bridge over a canal connecting two lakes. The lake on the right offers a short beach for dog swimming. On the left, the River Rock Trail joins the trail again. On the northeast shore of the dog-friendly lake, the Greenway Trail turns to the north, while the Mound Trail turns to the south—take that grassy trail. Hike along with a clear view of the lake to the west; continue straight ahead to the tree row and take the small loop trail to the left to view the American Indian mound. An interpretive sign explains its significance.

The Mound Trail ends at 1.9 miles at a road crossing at the picnic shelter. On the opposite side of the road, the route becomes the Lake View Trail. This path is mowed grass until it reaches the bridle trail coming in on the left from Amity Road. Lake View Trail follows the lakeshore and offers several points to pause and observe largemouth bass and sunfish cruising in the clear water. Watch your step on this trail, as it is shared with horses, and what horses drop as they travel along.

The Lake View Trail ends at the bridge, which you previously used to cross the Big Darby. The Alder Trail heads south from this point, following the creek and then passing through a meadow. Follow this narrow, packed-dirt trail, watching out for roots and stones. At 3.1 miles the Alder Trail meets the Sycamore Plains Trail. This path is composed of three trails: Sycamore Plains, Osage Opening, and the Tallgrass. The trail enters the woods from the meadow and splits— take the left option and traverse a woodland hillside to arrive at the parking area accessed from Amity Road.

The Sycamore Plains Trail continues south from near the parking area and follows the wood's edge. A couple of hundred feet along the trail, find the Tallgrass Trail and interpretive sign on the left. Remain on the Sycamore Trail to enter the woods and carefully descend a narrow, muddy path to the Big Darby. At the creek, the Osage Opening Trail leads away to the left and makes a 0.5-mile loop through the forest. This hike doesn't include this route, but it's an option if you have extra time. The Sycamore Trail follows the Big

Darby upstream, through riparian forest cover, before returning to the Alder Trail.

Retrace the path on the Alder Trail for 0.5 mile to return to the bridge and cross the Big Darby. Then turn left and follow the Bridle Trail south for about 100 yards. The Bridle Trail continues straight; instead, turn right at the Coneflower Trail intersection. Continue southwest on the midsection of the Coneflower, not taking either of the Coneflower north or south loops, for about 0.1 mile to meet the Darby Creek Greenway Trail. Turn north, passing through a field, and take the next left, which leads to the Whispering Oaks parking area. Look up and you might spy a red-tailed hawk soaring over the restored meadow in search of its next meal.

Nearby Attractions

About 5 miles northeast of the park is another, but much smaller, Metro Park—Heritage Trail. A paved 7-mile rails-to-trails multiuse corridor runs through the park. It continues in a straight line beginning at the historic district of Hilliard and ending in Plain City. The "Old Hilliard" section offers shopping, dining, and village parks to complete the trip to the prairie lands of western Franklin County.

Directions

From west of I-270 on I-70, take Exit 85 and travel north on Plain City–Georgesville Road for 0.8 mile to the park entrance on the right.

9

Sharon Woods
Metro Park

SCENERY: ★ ★ ★
TRAIL CONDITION: ★ ★ ★ ★ ★
CHILDREN: ★ ★ ★ ★ ★
DIFFICULTY: ★
SOLITUDE: ★ ★

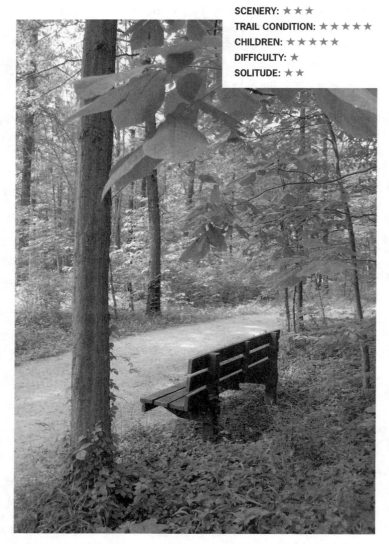

TAKE A SEAT AND OBSERVE THE WOODLAND RESIDENTS CROSSING THE TRAIL.

GPS TRAILHEAD COORDINATES: N40° 06.684' W82° 57.775'

DISTANCE & CONFIGURATION: 1.4-mile loop

HIKING TIME: About 1 hour

HIGHLIGHTS: Large oak trees, old fields, observation deck

ELEVATION: 849' at trailhead; 738' to 899' overall

ACCESS: Winter and fall, 6:30 a.m.–8 p.m.; summer, 6:30 a.m.–10 p.m.

MAPS: Bulletin board on side of naturalist office; **tinyurl.com/sharonwoods**

FACILITIES: Restrooms, drinking water, picnic areas, fishing pond
(15 and younger, 60 and older)

WHEELCHAIR ACCESS: Yes

COMMENTS: Highways border two sides of the park, so expect some road noise during
the hike.

CONTACTS: 6911 Cleveland Avenue, Westerville, OH 43081; 614-891-0700;
tinyurl.com/sharonwoods

Overview

Old-growth oaks and beech trees stand tall among the mixed deciduous
forest, shading the Edward S. Thomas Trail in the park's southwestern
quarter. The selected side route, the Oak Openings Trail, features
remnants of old fields still evident in the forest. A wooden boardwalk
leads out to an observation deck overlooking a field covered with tall
vegetation during midsummer. The hike ends at a fishing lake where
you can watch the largemouth bass swimming along the dock.

Route Details

You'll find plenty of natural diversity at this 760-acre park, and
it's highlighted at the Edward S. Thomas Preserve, named for a
well-known and respected naturalist and also one of Metro Parks'
founding board members. People like Thomas, who envisioned the
need to preserve natural areas, have been battling the ill effects of
urban sprawl for decades—and winning for the public's sake. The
sound of the highways bordering the park may be a constant, but the
abundance of interesting trees and other living things finding refuge
in the woods keeps your attention.

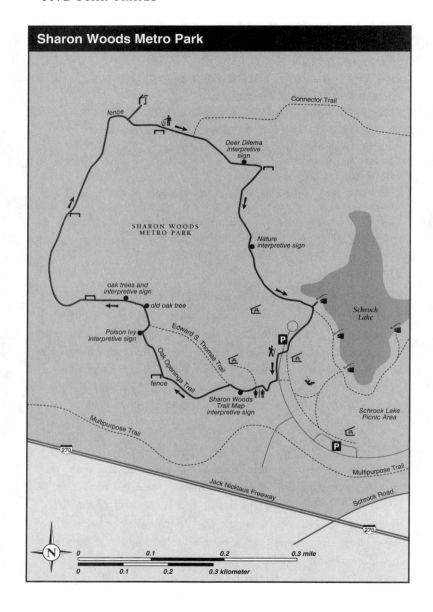

Sharon Woods Metro Park

Connector Trail

fence

Deer Dilema
interpretive
sign

Nature
interpretive sign

SHARON WOODS
METRO PARK

Schrock
Lake

oak trees and
interpretive sign

old oak tree

Poison Ivy
interpretive sign

Edward S. Thomas Trail

Oak Openings Trail

fence

Sharon Woods
Trail Map
interpretive sign

Schrock Lake
Picnic Area

Multipurpose Trail

270

Multipurpose Trail

Jack Nicklaus Freeway

Schrock Road

270

N

| 0 | 0.1 | 0.2 | 0.3 mile |

| 0 | 0.1 | 0.2 | 0.3 kilometer |

The trailhead is near the restroom on the left as you drive into the Schrock Lake parking area. A wide lawn includes four picnic shelters, playgrounds, and dozens of shade trees. Most picnickers linger in this area, with only a few following the Edward S. Thomas Trail into the forest. After just a few yards, you may feel you have the place to yourself—even in the middle of the day. As you start, notice the drinking water fountain near the restroom. It's not that the trail is physically demanding and extra water is a necessity, but the fountain is a welcome convenience. A couple of yards beyond the restroom on the 8-foot-wide trail, a paved path sneaks off to the right and leads to a picnic shelter. Stay on the main trail and you'll arrive at an interpretive sign introducing you to the Edward S. Thomas Preserve and the Sharon Woods trail map. At 0.1 mile the Oak Openings Trail turns off to the left—follow that.

The Oak Openings Trail adds approximately 0.25 mile to our hike. It stays in the forest, passing by a few small meadows. Watch out for a short strand of rusty fence wire protruding from a tree trunk, remnants of the farms that thrived here a century ago. A trailside bench invites you to pause at 0.2 mile, and across the trail from the bench you'll see a small field with an army of sapling trees

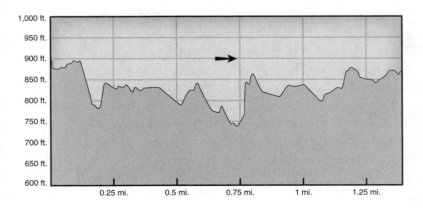

surrounding its perimeter, trying to reclaim the opening for the forest. If you sit here during the first couple of hours after sunrise, expect to see a deer or even a wild turkey foraging in the field. During rainy times, water pools throughout the forest, but the raised trail bed does not flood. The woodland wetlands come alive in the spring with peepers and spotted salamanders. At 0.3 mile the Oak Openings Trail rejoins the Edward S. Thomas Trail.

One hundred feet down the trail from the convergence stands a huge oak tree that has seen a couple hundred years of human presence. The old tree makes you wonder what the place was like 200 years prior. One thing's for sure—no highway noise or passenger jets flying overhead. On the trail, 120 feet ahead, are five large oak trees standing in a line. Likely growing at a field edge many years ago, the trees now reside deep in the forest. The woods are healthy with an active ecosystem in action—decaying trees on the ground and living trees supporting the canopy. Although there's not much in the way of wildflower displays, what the forest walk is missing in a colorful carpet, it gains in an impressive show of old trees that keep you looking up in awe. At 0.4 mile an interpretive sign on the right titled TRAVEL BACK IN TIME gives some insight into the various cultures that called this park home over the past several thousand years.

The trail bends around a right turn and heads north. This stretch of trail resembles an old, narrow country lane bordered by large-trunked trees on both sides. As it turns to the east, following a quarter-mile straight stretch, you'll see the access path and boardwalk to the observation deck on the left—0.75 mile from your vehicle. The elevated 30-foot wooden structure offers access to wheelchairs and strollers. From the observation deck, a 180-degree view of a meadow reveals not only wildlife, but also glimpses of hikers cruising past on the opposite side of the meadow. A pleasant breeze usually flows across the field and over the deck, adding another element to please the senses.

At the 0.9-mile mark, the connector trail from the Spring Creek Trail intersects your path from the left, but you stay straight on the Edward S. Thomas Trail. For the next 0.2 mile, a younger forest hosts the walk. The trail leaves the woods and enters a brushy field at 1.2 miles. A split rail fence, which serves as a perch for birds and dragonflies busily filling their two-month life span, follows the left side of the trail. One hundred yards ahead, the stone-and-dirt hiking trail meets the paved sidewalks of the picnic area. Schrock Lake is off to the left, and the parking lot where you began this hike is on the right.

Nearby Attractions

Two Metro Parks are nearby: Highbanks is 3 miles to the northwest, and Blendon Woods is to the southeast. The popular Polaris area bordering the northern stretches of the park offers a plethora of dining, shopping, and entertainment possibilities.

Directions

From I-270 Exit 27, follow Cleveland Avenue north for 0.5 mile to the park entrance on the left.

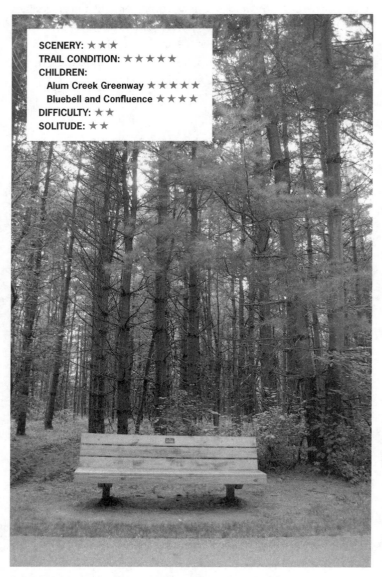

SCENERY: ★ ★ ★
TRAIL CONDITION: ★ ★ ★ ★ ★
CHILDREN:
  Alum Creek Greenway ★ ★ ★ ★ ★
  Bluebell and Confluence ★ ★ ★ ★
DIFFICULTY: ★ ★
SOLITUDE: ★ ★

A BENCH IN THE PINES TREATS RESTING HIKERS TO A FULFILLMENT
OF THE SENSES.

GPS TRAILHEAD COORDINATES: N39° 52.840' W82° 54.208'

DISTANCE & CONFIGURATION: 3.1-mile figure eight

HIKING TIME: About 2.5 hours

HIGHLIGHTS: Creeks, riparian forest

ELEVATION: 762' at trailhead, with no significant rise

ACCESS: April–September: daily, 6:30 a.m.–10 p.m.; October–March, daily, 6:30 a.m.–8 p.m.

MAPS: At bulletin boards, **tinyurl.com/threecreeks**

FACILITIES: Restrooms, drinking water, picnic areas, playground, Natural Play Area

WHEELCHAIR ACCESS: Yes, on Alum Creek Greenway

COMMENTS: The creek trails are subject to closure during high water periods. Chain gates and warning signs will alert visitors if trails are impassable.

CONTACTS: 3860 Bixby Road, Groveport, OH 43125; 614-891-0700; **tinyurl.com/threecreeks**

Overview

For millions of us, playing in a creek was the first time we discovered nature. Three Creeks Metro Park's waterways and surrounding natural areas attract guests of all ages wanting to reconnect with the natural world. Bluebell and Confluence Trails explore the banks and views of Alum and Blacklick Creeks as they join the Big Walnut Creek heading south. Cross the Big Walnut on a steel bridge on the paved, multiuse Alum Creek Greenway Trail, which covers half the mileage for this hike.

Route Details

Although located within a mile of Interstate 270, this Metro Park pulls visitors into a natural state, benefiting both body and mind. For kids, the park has one of the Metro Park System's great Natural Play Areas. From the parking lot where the hike starts, young ones can enter the 12-acre pine forest to climb trees, flip over logs in search of critters, or see what they can discover in the carpet of fallen pine needles. These areas were created to provide a real connection with the natural world for a generation of kids from an electronic world.

Three Creeks Metro Park

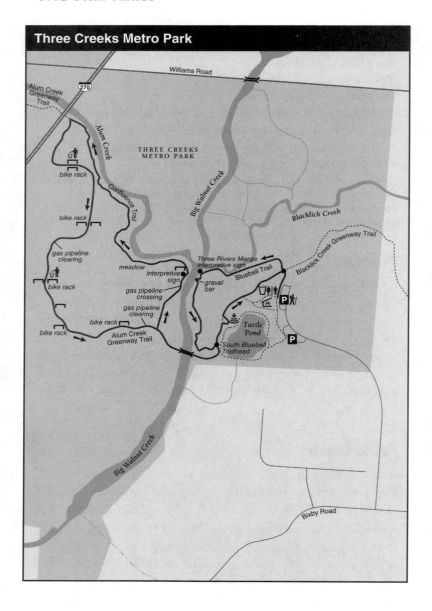

The Confluence Trails Area is a popular picnic spot for families at this 1,050-acre park. Visitors can explore various landscapes on 14 miles of trails, but the most interesting feature at Three Creeks is, well, the creeks—and their confluence. The Bluebell Trail trailhead is found at the edge of the lawn north of the parking lot. In just a few steps, the Bluebell Trail changes from park atmosphere to natural creek bottom. At this trailhead and three others providing gateways to the creeks, you'll find chain gates with metal signs warning of the danger of high water. If the chain gate is open, the trails are open. If the gates are closed, stay out for your own safety. Don't ignore the warnings. You may consider the creeks shallow and harmless, but they can swell and run over their banks surprisingly quickly.

Large trees with large canopies shade the creek bank, so enjoy cool hiking during the spring and summer. In the fall, expect a colorful display of leaves decorating the creek bottoms. Huge sycamores populate both sides of the creeks throughout the entire hike. Cottonwood trees are equally big, and when the breeze blows their leaves flutter like aspen, adding another soothing sound to the creekside hike. Along the Bluebell Trail, easy access points allow you to get close to Blacklick Creek. But the star location at the park and

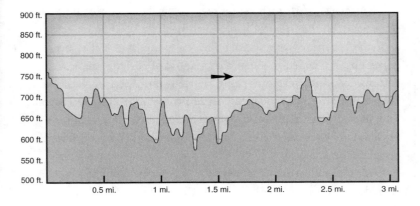

its namesake are just ahead. At 0.4 mile you'll find an interpretive sign—and the confluence of Blacklick and Alum Creeks with Big Walnut Creek.

On the Bluebell Trail side of the confluence, a large gravel bar stretches out into the creek. A short spur trail spills out onto the gravel bar; this is a great spot for taking photos up- and downstream, unless the water is running a bit high—just use common sense. During late summer, a buckeye tree a few steps downstream from the gravel bar lowers its branches toward the trail with its fruit hidden inside a tan, round pod with tiny, spiky bumps. The Bluebell Trail completes its creek tour at 0.6 mile and curves up out of the creek gully to meet the Alum Creek Greenway Trail, a paved, multiuse path.

Turn right (west) and cross the iron-and-wood bridge over Big Walnut Creek, taking in nice views up and down the waterway. During wildflower season, a good showing of color appears around the short meadow on the southwest side of the bridge. One-tenth of a mile from the bridge, on the north side of the paved trail, you'll reach the second creekside route of this hike, the Confluence Trail. A pine grove welcomes you to the west side of the creeks for about 100 yards. The Confluence Trail seems to get the least amount of foot traffic, so if you'd like a brief moment of quietude, you may be in luck.

After a westerly turn in the creek, you will reach the confluence once again, but on the west bank this time. Here you'll find another sign and a bench. Working your way west, the creek riffles over a gravel bottom, emitting the pleasant sound of moving water. More cottonwoods and sycamores stand tall along both sides of the creek. The stroll from the confluence north to the end of the Confluence Trail flanks Alum Creek. During warm months, add a bottle of insect repellent to your day pack. Mosquitoes and other biting insects populate the creek.

At 1.6 miles the Confluence Trail emerges from the creek's shoulder and joins the Alum Creek Greenway Trail. I-270 hums by a dozen yards north of this trail junction. Turn left (south) and commence your return hike on the paved pathway as it passes by two aquatic study ponds and through a woodland. Six sets of benches and bike racks are spread out trailside on the way back to the bridge. At 2.2 miles you'll find a wooden bench in front of a grove of white pines facing a young forest. Sit and listen. The drone of the interstate is replaced with singing birds and insects. From the Big Walnut Creek bridge, you have 0.5 mile to go to your vehicle. Watch for the frequent bicyclists who also use the paved trail.

Nearby Attractions

The newest park in the Columbus Metro Park system, Walnut Woods, is located about 3 miles southeast of Three Creeks. The new park is primarily in the development stage, but sections opened in 2012, and in the previous year, the Tall Pines Area debuted with 2.5 miles of paved trail. The central section of the park is scheduled to open in 2013. The Tall Pines Area is located at 6833 Richardson Road, Groveport, OH 43125.

Directions

From I-270, take US 33 southeast for 1.1 miles. Turn right on Hamilton Road and travel south 1.5 miles to Bixby Road and turn right. The park entrance is on the right in 1.2 miles.

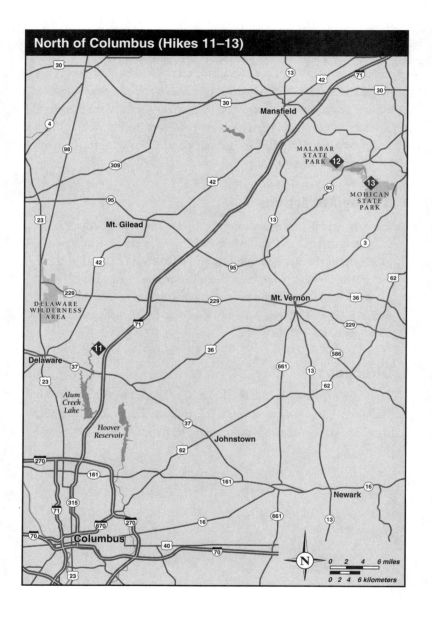

North of Columbus (Hikes 11–13)

North

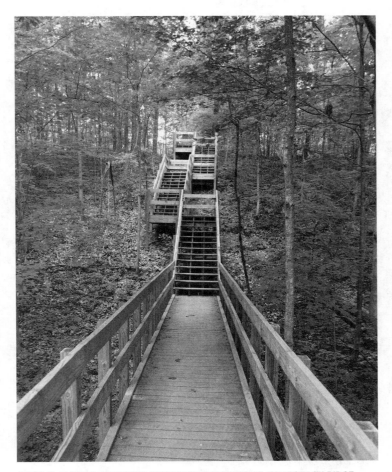

SEVERAL FLIGHTS OF STAIRS GET THE HEART PUMPING AT HOGBACK RIDGE.

Hogback Ridge Preserve

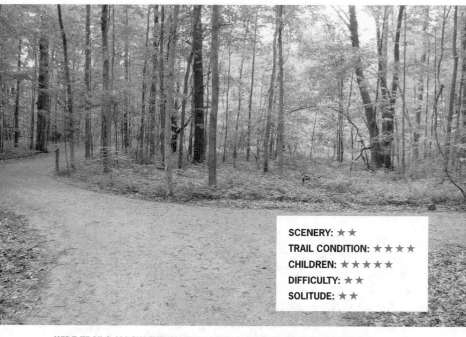

SCENERY: ★ ★
TRAIL CONDITION: ★ ★ ★ ★
CHILDREN: ★ ★ ★ ★ ★
DIFFICULTY: ★ ★
SOLITUDE: ★ ★

WIDE TRAILS ALLOW THE FAMILY TO WALK SIDE BY SIDE, HAND IN HAND.

GPS TRAILHEAD COORDINATES: N40° 18.615' W82° 56.403'

DISTANCE & CONFIGURATION: 1.1-mile loop

HIKING TIME: About 1 hour

HIGHLIGHTS: Ravine crossing, pond/wildlife blind

ELEVATION: 987' at trailhead; 819' to 986' overall

ACCESS: Year-round, 8 a.m.–sunset

MAPS: Nature center, bulletin board at parking area, **tinyurl.com/hogbackridge**

FACILITIES: Picnic area, restrooms, drinking water, comprehensive nature center

WHEELCHAIR ACCESS: Yes, but not paved on the Woodland Ridge Trail

COMMENTS: Ravine crossing includes more than 80 stair steps.

CONTACTS: 2656 Hogback Road, Sunbury, OH 43074; 740-524-8600;
tinyurl.com/hogbackridge

Overview

Two trails, Woodland Ridge and Pinegrove, lead hikers through two primary forest environments, deciduous and evergreen. The loops are linked with a ravine crossing on a 40-foot wooden bridge, and a set of stairs on each side of the ravine. The two loops are easy walking (with little elevation change), and the crushed limestone trails are well groomed. At the southern point of the Pinegrove Trail, a wood wall with viewing slots provides a fun wildlife blind along a pond. At the end of the hike, the Mary Barber McCoy Nature Center offers multiple displays with interpretive signage. The nature center is open Monday–Friday, 9 a.m.–4 p.m.; weekends and holidays, noon–5 p.m.

Route Details

Delaware County is experiencing urban sprawl. But the county's Preservation Parks system, which has a mission of providing recreation with minimal development, is trying to combat the loss of natural areas, and you can see some of its work here.

As soon as you exit your vehicle in the wooded parking area, you'll feel a calming sense of connection with nature. The Woodland Ridge Trail leaves and returns from the nature center, and this is where we will start our hike. From the parking area's northern stretch, look to the west for a sign identifying the Woodland Ridge Trail. The 10-foot-wide path welcomes you to the hardwood forest with a mature shagbark hickory tree being the first to greet you. Three hundred feet into the hike the first of several tree identification signs appears trailside. This one is devoted to the black cherry tree. To the right and down a steep 50-foot slope, a small stream trickles along a gully floor.

The trail continues west along the ridge with various hardwood tree species intermixed, creating a pleasant forest scene. You'll feel lucky to be walking there. After 0.2 mile you'll see the first of a few trailside benches offering the chance to sit and listen to the woodland and its small creatures scurrying under and over the carpet of leaf

Hogback Ridge Preserve

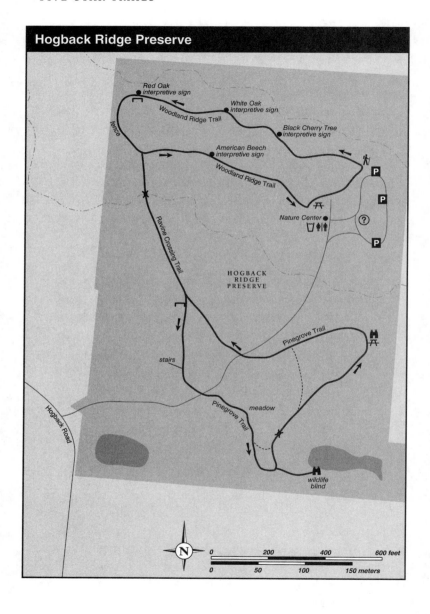

Red Oak
interpretive sign

White Oak
interpretive sign

Black Cherry Tree
interpretive sign

Woodland Ridge Trail

American Beech
interpretive sign

Woodland Ridge Trail

fence

Nature Center

Ravine Crossing Trail

HOGBACK
RIDGE
PRESERVE

Pinegrove Trail

stairs

Pinegrove Trail

meadow

Hogback Road

wildlife
blind

N

0   200   400   600 feet

0   50   100   150 meters

litter. Children will want to spend some time and try to spot one of the little critters making all the noise. The trail turns to the left (the Woodland Ridge Trail is only 0.4 mile) and heads south. The Ravine Crossing Trail, which is also the connecting trail of the two loops, turns off to the right—take this trail. The wooden staircases and footbridge at the bottom of the ravine appear right away. You will return to this point on the way back.

The approximately 40 wooden steps leading down to the bridge are mirrored on the opposite side of the ravine. The creek passing under the bridge is alive with minnows that school up in the holes in the creek bottom. Pause here for a few minutes to gather the energy to climb the stairs up and out of the ravine, and while re-energizing, watch and listen for a pileated woodpecker—a resident of the preserve. After making the climb up the stairs, you'll meet the Pinegrove Trail. Turn right (south) to begin the second loop of the hike and the preserve. A set of wood-framed steps filled with crushed limestone leads up a rise in the grove at 0.4 mile. The remainder of the Pinegrove Trail is void of any steps. One hundred feet ahead is the first park road crossing. Although autos should be traveling less

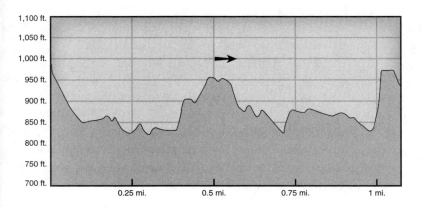

than 15 mph, watch out for traffic and rejoin the trail as it enters a mix of pines and deciduous trees.

After traveling 150 feet from the road crossing, the trail meets a small, open brushy field, and then turns quickly to the left. A spur runs off to the right as the trail turns—follow that to the wildlife blind on the edge of a secluded pond. It has several viewing slots cut into the wall at different heights and will accommodate even the shortest wildlife watcher. During spring and summer, scan the logs in and along the pond for turtles sunning themselves. Pause at the blind long enough and you may see a wood duck landing on the water. If you think you'd like to stay here awhile, strap a folding stool to your pack for more comfortable sitting.

You'll reenter the grove about 100 feet from the spur trail point. Dame's rockets in various shades of purple stand along the trail during the spring, providing a colorful wildflower show on the floor of the pine grove. At 0.6 mile, a bench offers a rest and a great view of the preserve's wooded ravine. The trail re-crosses the park road and leads through a stand of young hickory trees before returning to the Ravine Crossing Trail. Turn right and cross the ravine via the 80 steps and the bridge to arrive back on the Woodland Ridge Trail. Your workout is nearly complete. Turn right on the Woodland Ridge Trail and hike the last 0.1 mile to the nature center. It's a must-visit if it's open, featuring extensive displays of the woodland environment you just explored. *Note:* As an option, a less-ambitious hiker can join you on a portion of this hike, but remain on the Woodland Ridge Trail, avoiding the ravine, stairs, bridge, and road crossings.

Nearby Attractions

Alum Creek State Park is less than 1 mile from the preserve. Alum Creek reservoir provides more than 3,000 acres of water for boating, fishing, and swimming at Ohio's largest inland beach. Hoover Reservoir is a short drive to the southeast and also a popular destination. A third large body of water, Delaware Lake in Delaware

State Park, is located northwest of Alum Creek State Park. For some friendly competition, give disc golf a try at the state parks. The sport has become quite popular over the past couple of years.

Directions

From Columbus, take I-71 north for 23 miles to Exit 131. Turn west and go 0.7 mile to CR 35 on the right. Travel north 1.5 miles to Howard Road on the left. Go 0.5 mile to Hogback Road on the right and drive 1.25 miles to the preserve entrance on the right.

Malabar Farm
State Park

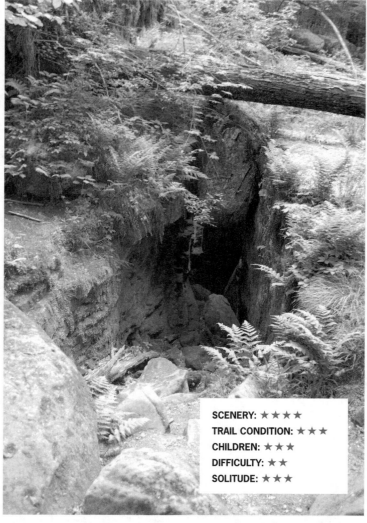

SCENERY: ★ ★ ★ ★
TRAIL CONDITION: ★ ★ ★
CHILDREN: ★ ★ ★
DIFFICULTY: ★ ★
SOLITUDE: ★ ★ ★

SEVERAL ROCK CREVICES CREATED BY THOUSANDS OF YEARS OF EROSION ARE
FOUND TRAILSIDE.

GPS TRAILHEAD COORDINATES: N40° 39.095' W82° 23.580'

DISTANCE & CONFIGURATION: 1.6-mile balloon

HIKING TIME: About 1 hour

HIGHLIGHTS: Cave, rock outcropping, living farm displays

ELEVATION: 1,115' at trailhead, 940' to 1,267' overall

ACCESS: Closes at sunset; no fees or permits required

MAPS: At park's visitor center, bulletin board at trailhead parking, **malabarfarm.org**

FACILITIES: Restroom at visitor center

WHEELCHAIR ACCESS: No

COMMENTS: Crevices between rocks above falls are approachable on foot, but exercise caution.

CONTACTS: 4050 Bromfield Road, Lucas, OH 44843; 419-892-2784; **malabarfarm.org**

Overview

The hike starts at a working farm with extensive agricultural displays from the past and present, which are worth a visit after hiking. A walk up a gravel lane from the farm is required to reach the start of the Butternut Trail, one of three paths on the property. You'll pass by a remote cabin and outbuildings at the start of the actual trail, and soon arrive at a small sandstone cave with a boulder field above it, prime for exploring. Loop around the top of a wooded ridge before returning to the cabin in the woods.

Route Details

Pleasant Valley, home to Malabar Farm State Park, has captured the attention of naturalists, farmers, and a Pulitzer Prize–winning author for nearly a century. The writer and conservationist, Louis Bromfield, built the farm's 32-room house in 1939—it's now a national historic site. Its impressive agricultural displays and interpretive programs will likely pull you in before and after you explore the ridge to the south via the Butternut Trail. For a panoramic view of the farm and the Pleasant Valley expanse, follow signs to the peak of Mt. Jeez, just east of the state park entrance on Pleasant Valley Road.

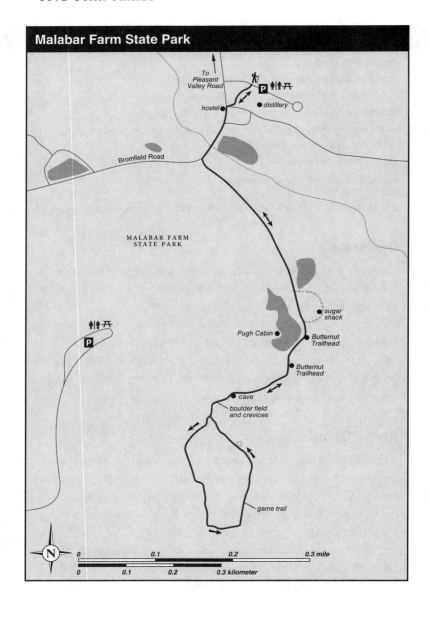

Malabar Farm State Park

To Pleasant Valley Road

hostel

distillery

Bromfield Road

MALABAR FARM STATE PARK

sugar shack

Pugh Cabin

Butternut Trailhead

Butternut Trailhead

cave

boulder field and crevices

game trail

N

| 0 | | 0.1 | | 0.2 | | 0.3 mile |
| 0 | 0.1 | | 0.2 | | 0.3 kilometer | |

Several parking areas dot the grounds, but you'll start this hike from the paved lot on the left side of Bromfield Road; it's just to the right after passing the entrance to the visitor center. A few barns and tilled displays adjoin this lot. After cinching up your boot strings, walk between the barn and machinery shed and down the gravel lot toward the pond. Continue past the picnic area at the pond's north bank and onto Bromfield Road. A hostel sits across the road and is usually occupied. Watch your step, as dozens of geese and ducks waddle around the barn areas and lots, but don't hesitate to talk to the friendly fowl.

Walk along the road's left berm for about 0.1 mile, crossing Switzer Run, a stream flowing over a shale and sandstone bed. Road traffic is fairly light, and even when it's a bit busier during the summer, drivers travel this stretch slowly because of the many people and animal crossing. Ten yards after the stream, turn left onto the gravel lane. A sign notes it's for emergency and authorized vehicles only, which is why you parked in the lot and are now walking up the gravel lane to reach the trailhead. At the beginning of the gravel lane, the Doris Duke Nature Trail loop, marked by blue blazes, takes off to the right, and can be an addition to your Malabar hiking adventure

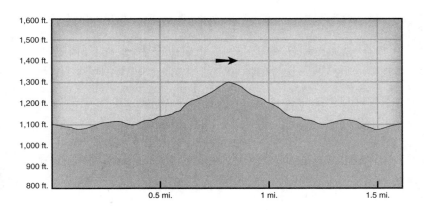

if you'd like. Continue up the lane for 0.3 mile, passing a pond and a maple syruping shack on the left, to reach the Butternut Trail and the Pugh Cabin, a day-use rental facility. It's surrounded by towering hemlocks, and it all blends to make a beautiful scene. A couple of yards from the sidewalk to the Pugh Cabin, you'll find the Butternut Trail sign and the start of the hike.

A two-car-sized boulder greets hikers as they start up the yellow-blazed trail. The big rock offers a hint of what lies ahead and what the glaciers left behind. The path is packed soil with many tree roots. Look downhill to see a small outbuilding behind the cabin—one end is built over an exposed boulder. When the owner, James Pugh, constructed the structure, he intended to remove the boulder. After digging, he found what were likely American Indian bones, so he reburied them and chose to leave the stone out of respect.

At 0.6 mile you arrive at the highlight of the trail—a narrow 16-foot-high cave only accessible by small animals. Maneuver up and around the left side of the cave to a boulder field. Fractures in the huge rocks have created crevices approximately 20 feet deep and a few feet wide. It's tough to avoid the urge to explore here, so watch your step.

One hundred feet up the trail from the boulder field, the trail splits—go right, although either way will loop back around to the point. The 0.4-mile loop ascends to nearly the top of a wooded ridge, rolling through various ages and species of hardwood trees. It's quiet up on the ridge except for the tweets and whistles of native songbirds, and it's no wonder that Bromfield enjoyed walks in these woods above his farmland. As the loop hits its peak and begins to descend, a few heavily used game trails intersect the hiking path. If you'd like to see wildlife, try this trail early in the morning. You may catch white-tailed deer working their way through the woods toward bedding areas after a night of feeding along the field edges. At 0.9 mile the trail turns muddy for a few yards because of an overly active spring. You'll arrive at the point where you began the loop, 300 feet ahead. Once back at the Pugh Cabin, take a seat along the lane and feel the spirit of this peaceful park before heading down the lane to the farm.

Nearby Attractions

Mohican Memorial State Forest and Mohican State Park are 7 miles southeast of Malabar and together provide nearly 6,000 acres of wild beauty to explore by foot, canoe or kayak, mountain bike, or on horseback. The region's primary attraction is Clear Fork Gorge and the Clear Fork River that runs through it. Mohican is one of Ohio's premier vacation destinations, with plenty of outdoors adventure for all ages. For boaters, Pleasant Hill Lake, 6 miles to the east, harbors a full-service marina, with rentals from pontoon boats to kayaks.

Directions

From Columbus, take I-71 north for 61 miles to Exit 169. Drive east 1.8 miles on Hanley Road. Turn right on Washington South Road and travel south 0.3 mile to a Y in the road. Take the left option, which is Pleasant Valley Road, and follow it 5.5 miles to the park entrance on the right.

13

Mohican State Park

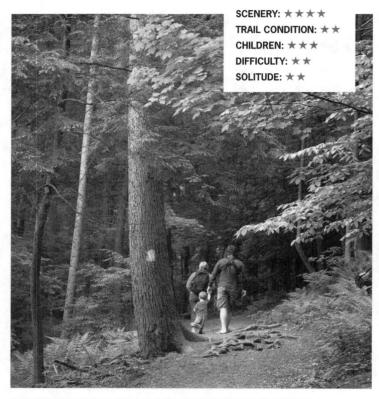

SCENERY: ★ ★ ★ ★
TRAIL CONDITION: ★ ★
CHILDREN: ★ ★ ★
DIFFICULTY: ★ ★
SOLITUDE: ★ ★

A YOUNG FAMILY FOLLOWS A BLAZED TRAIL THROUGH THE FOREST.

GPS TRAILHEAD COORDINATES: N40° 36.780' W82° 19.011'

DISTANCE & CONFIGURATION: 2.4-mile balloon

HIKING TIME: About 2 hours

HIGHLIGHTS: River's edge access and views, waterfalls

ELEVATION: 978' at trailhead; 674' to 1,123' overall

ACCESS: Closes at sunset; no fees or permits required

MAPS: At bulletin board at trailhead and **mohicanstatepark.org**

FACILITIES: Restrooms, picnic area with water sources on east side of covered bridge

WHEELCHAIR ACCESS: No

COMMENTS: Trail leads to Little Lyons Falls, with no safety barriers—keep children at hand.

CONTACTS: 419-994-5125; **mohicanstatepark.org**

Overview

Several trails provide access to an impressive gorge that will engage all of the senses. But Lyons Falls Trail includes everything that makes the gorge such a natural attraction—boreal-type forest, scenic river, waterfalls, and rock outcroppings. The Clear Fork of the Mohican River parallels the trail with several opportunities to get down to the water. After spying a brown trout feeding in the river, follow the trail up into a wide and deep ravine cradling a tributary to the Clear Fork. At the head of this gorge—and at the neighboring ravine to the north—water falls over a recessed cave, giving the trail its name.

Route Details

Mohican State Park and State Forest are popular with Ohioans. Picnickers by the dozens line up along the Clear Fork, downstream from a well-maintained covered bridge. The span finds its way into thousands of family photos each year, and rightly so—it's truly picturesque. Just to the south of the picnic area (on the northeast side of the river and covered bridge) is the primitive Class B campground. Staying a night along the banks of the Clear Fork after experiencing the gorge on foot is icing on the cake. Just don't forget to bring your fly rod and a handful of flies to catch a trout for dinner.

You'll find a paved roadside parking area near the covered bridge on the right. On weekends the dozen spaces may be taken, but simply drive across the bridge and turn right to find additional spots at the picnic area. It's common to pass picnickers on the trails, but only for the first mile or so on the way to Big Lyons Falls. Across the road from the parking area first noted, you'll find the trailhead by a double bulletin board and a couple of benches where you can sit and tighten boot strings before setting out. To the right of the trail, down a 40-foot slope, the river flows under the bridge. This area sees many waders and rock skippers, but hold back the urge to get wet here—there's ample space and time up the trail.

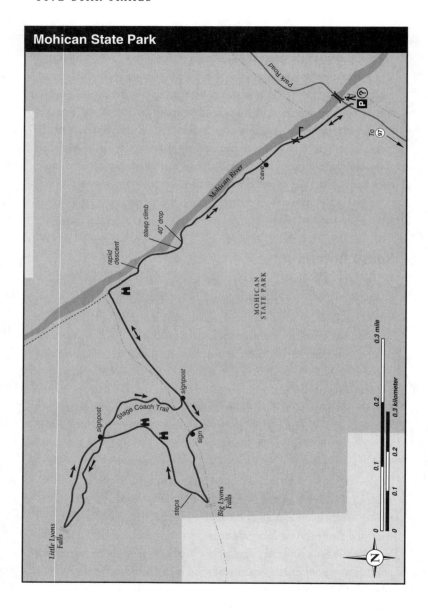

Mohican State Park

Dozens of small springs trickle down the hill, which muddies up the dirt trail at several points throughout this hike. However, wooden footbridges span the wettest and deepest spring runs. The first of these bridges and boardwalks is found at the 0.1-mile mark, accompanied by a wooden bench for four. The aroma of the mature hemlock trees and their bed of fallen needles fill the air with an intoxicating smell. White blazes keep you on track, but the well-worn dirt path is difficult to lose.

Watch your step, though, as the terrain shoots up and down and around tree roots and shallow holes and humps. But don't miss the non-stop scenery blanketing the gorge's floor and forested walls. If you've walked among the Great Smoky Mountains, this hike will remind you of that national park, thanks to the hemlock-dominated forest and associated woodland vegetation. At a few points along this riverside section of the trail, the forest squeezes the path down to only a couple of feet. The occasional downed tree temporarily allows sunlight to reach the forest floor, giving the undergrowth a chance to bush out.

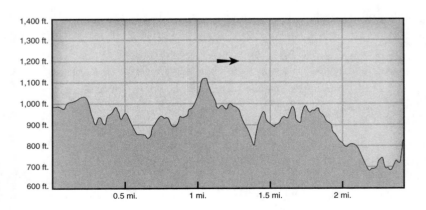

The Delaware Indians used the gorge and its river for hunting. Wildlife inhabited the valley centuries ago, and even today raccoons, deer, and wild turkeys roam here—go early in the morning to catch a glimpse of a deer drinking from the river's edge. At 0.5 mile the trail opens up, providing the option of a nearly level walk to the river and a wide gravel bar, or you can turn left and push up the ravine to Big Lyons Falls 0.5 mile ahead. You will be joined by jumping squirrels working their way up and down the ravine, providing a few laughs along the way. At 0.75 mile a signpost points to the Stage Coach Trail coming in on the right, which is the way to Little Lyons Falls and onward to Pleasant Hill Dam—you will pass here on your return trip of this balloon hike. For now, stay straight to reach Big Lyons Falls.

As the cascade comes into view, you'll hear the sound of a trickling creek falling 80 feet to a ravine floor. The trail leads to the heart of the falls, which is a recessed cave. Several 4-foot-square sandstone rocks sit near the spot where the water crashes to the ground; these rocks are popular for sitting and taking in the scenery. Studying the underside of the cave and falls will reveal dozens of small trees and fluffs of ferns growing from the seams in the rock, as if they are climbing up to find a bit more growing light. A layer of moss attempts to cover the graffiti carvings by thoughtless visitors. To get back to the hike, follow the incline up the right side of the cave opening. A set of wooden stairs takes you up and out of the gorge to continue on to Little Lyons Falls. At the top of those stairs, turn around (carefully) and gaze back at the falls for a nice photo op.

The trail heads east and rounds the side of the ridge separating the two waterfalls. Be careful: The path is narrow with a steep drop immediately off the edge. Just 0.25 mile from the top of the stairs, you'll find a signpost marking the way to the falls (straight) or turn right to take the Stage Coach Trail. Little Lyons Falls is 1.4 miles into the hike. This smaller falls is only a 25-foot drop, and the trail will take you to the top. There are no safety railings, so use common sense and take caution—especially with kids. The falls drops into a stone canyon, and from the top it's difficult to follow the water's progress unless you peek over the edge. The trail continues around and up the north side of the falls and proceeds to the dam. But average hikers should avoid this short climb, because if you slip, you'll likely slide over the falls. Turn around and return to the last signpost. Follow the Stage Coach Trail back to the main trail that you came in on and return to the covered bridge.

Nearby Attractions

The Loudonville-Mohican area is a busy vacation destination throughout the summer. An abundance of canoe liveries handle the packs of river runners that are a constant sight in the Clear Fork and Mohican Rivers. Mohican Memorial State Forest offers 4,500 additional acres of woodlands to explore and 32 additional miles of hiking trails. Mohican State Park's lodge overlooks Pleasant Hill Lake. Malabar Farm State Park is 7 miles to the northwest of Mohican State Park. The working-farm park (with tours) was the home of the famous author Louis Bromfield.

Directions

From Columbus, take I-71 north for 57 miles to Exit 165. Turn east on OH 97 and travel 16 miles to the park road (signage posted). Turn left and follow the park road 1.25 miles to the covered bridge.

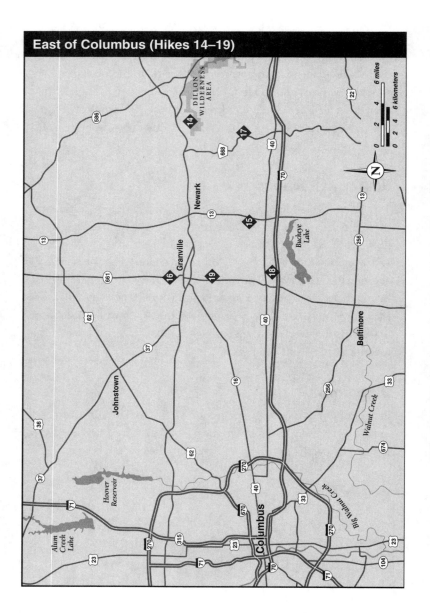

East of Columbus (Hikes 14–19)

East

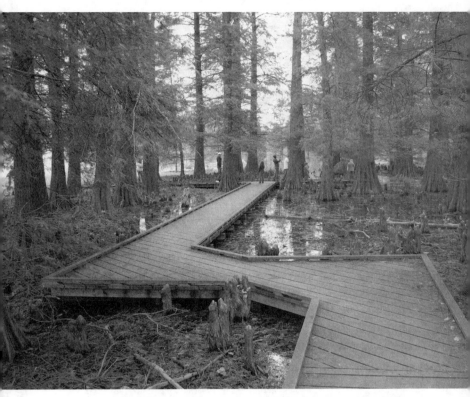

CYPRESS KNEES RISE UP FROM THE SWAMP SURROUNDING THE BOARDWALK.

14

Blackhand Gorge
State Nature Preserve

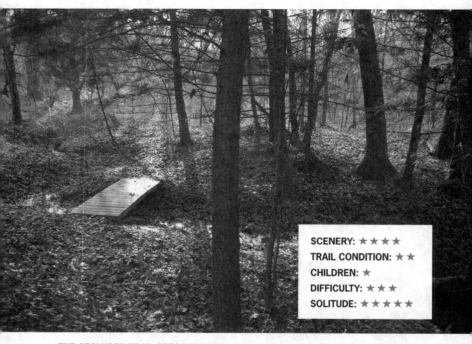

SCENERY: ★ ★ ★ ★
TRAIL CONDITION: ★ ★
CHILDREN: ★
DIFFICULTY: ★ ★ ★
SOLITUDE: ★ ★ ★ ★ ★

THE SECLUDED TRAIL SEES VERY LITTLE FOOT TRAFFIC OVER THIS FOOTBRIDGE.

GPS TRAILHEAD COORDINATES: N40° 03.522' W82° 14.300'

DISTANCE & CONFIGURATION: 2.5-mile loop

HIKING TIME: About 2 hours

HIGHLIGHTS: River vista, mature deciduous forest, bluff

ELEVATION: 845' at trailhead; 754' to 1,019' overall

ACCESS: Closes at sunset; no fees or permits required

MAPS: At parking area bulletin board and **tinyurl.com/blackhandgorgesnp**

FACILITIES: None

WHEELCHAIR ACCESS: No

COMMENTS: No pets allowed; trail passes near cliff edge—stay on trail.

CONTACTS: 614-265-6453; **tinyurl.com/blackhandgorgesnp**

Overview

Blackhand Gorge State Nature Preserve offers hikers two options—a level, paved roadway path and one that caters to the more adventurous. If you prefer solitude on the trail, then the Marie Hickey Trail is your best bet. It rambles over the hills and through the woods, providing views of distant ridges and peeks down 50-foot bluffs to the Licking River below. Add the short Oak Knob Trail and you have a complete set of woodland trails. The trail skirts along the top edges of ravines rich with wildlife. Go slowly so as not to spook the show.

Route Details

This nature preserve was created to protect the flora and fauna that thrive in and around the gorge cut by the Licking River. The preserve got its intriguing name because of a dark hand petroglyph that once decorated the gorge wall. Unfortunately, the marking was destroyed in the early 1800s during construction of the Ohio-Erie Canal. American Indian lore permeates this place, and after walking among the hills surrounding the natural feature, you'll feel it too.

The primary parking area and trailhead for the 4-mile-long, wide, paved Blackhand Trail is on the north side of the town of Toboso, along the south bank of the Licking River. The multiuse Blackhand Trail is the most popular hike at the gorge, running west from the main trailhead, with a few spurs for added hiking. On summer weekends, bicyclists and walkers create a steady flow of visitors throughout the day. Our trails, the Marie Hickey and Oak Knob, are on the north side of the Licking River and away from the crowds. However, if a physically challenged hiker or a child is joining you, go ahead and do the Blackhand Trail, as it does provide a great look at the gorge from the bottom.

From the north parking area, the Marie Hickey Trail leads off to the right of the bulletin board. The route tests your stamina right at the start as it shoots straight up the ridge toward the highest point of the hike. At 0.2 mile the trail passes a signpost with an arrow

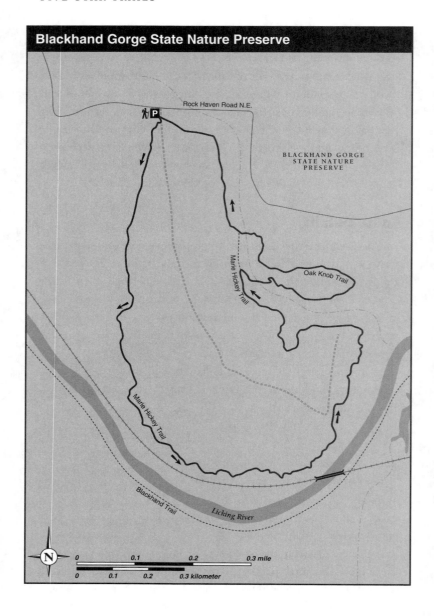

Blackhand Gorge State Nature Preserve

Rock Haven Road N.E.

BLACKHAND GORGE
STATE NATURE
PRESERVE

Oak Knob Trail

Marie Hickey Trail

Marie Hickey Trail

Blackhand Trail

Licking River

N

| 0 | 0.1 | 0.2 | 0.3 mile |
| 0 | 0.1 | 0.2 | 0.3 kilometer |

directing you to follow an oil well service dirt road, continuing the ascent. In summer this portion of the trail is kept cool by the tree canopy. Just 0.1 mile later, another arrowed signpost steers you off the dirt road and back onto the trail. During autumn, the trail becomes hard to find, hidden under a blanket of leaves. At 0.2 mile you will reach the peak of the tallest ridge and begin a slow, pleasant descent with views of neighboring ridges to the west. Sit on a log and admire the Appalachian foothills—your time will be well spent.

The landscape levels out somewhat and follows the upper edge of a stone bluff overlooking the Licking River and the Blackhand Trail 50 feet below and on the opposite side of the river. You can see and hear the patrons below on the paved path, but you remain less exposed on the forested cliff top. With great river views to the right, few think to look left. Those who do see a field surrounded by forest with young trees, wild shrubs, and the occasional oil pump jack. At 0.75 mile a stand of evergreens flanks the left side of the trail as it scoots closer to the cliff edge. A clear view of the river and railroad trestle appears 500 feet down the trail. Another 200 feet, and the trail and cliff edge are separated by only 8 feet. If a child is with you, hold his or her hand for safe passage. This is also the prime point

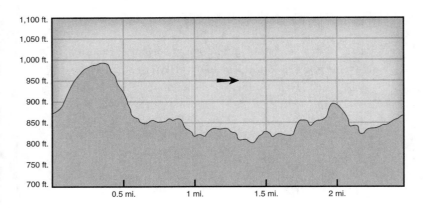

to capture a photo of the river below and the stone bluff and grand forest on the opposing bank.

At 1.1 miles the trail turns back north, away from the cliff edge, although the cliff eventually tapers off, leaving a minimal bank at the river. A shallow valley slopes up from the river and meets a meadow of mixed brush and scattered trees. Deer use this passage often, so you may have some wild company as you pass through. Travel 0.2 mile and take a last look at the river as the trail turns back into the forest. Look down the ravine to the right and see if you can spot a remnant of life here a century ago. *Hint:* A few concrete blocks and a portion of a brick chimney still stand. Throughout the rest of the hike, you will pass other signs of century- (or two) old dwellings between the ridges.

A group of hemlock trees comes into view straight ahead, looking a bit out of place with open hardwood forest surrounding them. As you get closer, the air temp drops a few degrees as the trail descends a bit and curves into the hemlocks. The trees stand at the head of a cut in the bedrock, forming a small gorge only several yards in depth and length, but a beautiful landform just the same. At the end of the little hemlock grove, the trail crosses a small bridge and moves along the opposite side of the little gorge. A few more steps and the trail drops into a shallow ravine that is crossed with a wooden bridge with a set of steps going up the other side. At 1.6 miles the trail passes over a sandstone outcropping, so watch your step. Just 0.1 mile more and Oak Knob Trail loops off to the right—take it.

Oak Knob Trail wanders around an oak-dominated ridge (hence the name) with a couple of stone ledges cantilevered out over the ravine. After touring the ridge for 0.6 mile, you rejoin the primary trail farther north than where you left it. The last 0.3 mile shoots straight through a mowed path in the center of a field of dense brush. Multiple game trails intersect, so peek over your shoulder occasionally for a photo op.

Nearby Attractions

To the southeast of the preserve is Dillon State Park, which offers mountain bike, equestrian, multiuse, and hiking trails. Seven picnic areas with great views of the lake are available. Boat-launching ramps and a modern campground also await outdoors enthusiasts.

Directions

From Columbus, take OH 16 for 43 miles through Newark to OH 146. Turn south on OH 146 and travel 0.2 mile. Turn right on Toboso Road and drive south 1.3 miles. Turn right on Rock Haven Road and travel west 1 mile to the parking area on the left.

Dawes Arboretum

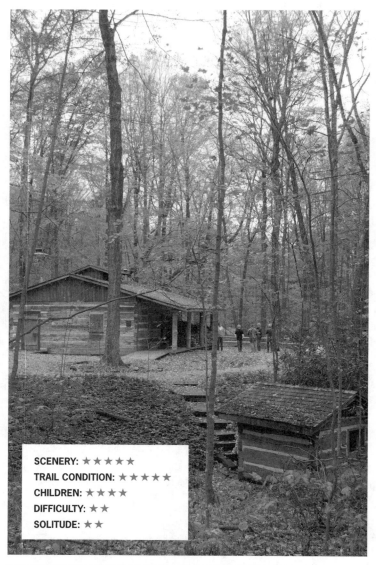

SCENERY: ★ ★ ★ ★ ★
TRAIL CONDITION: ★ ★ ★ ★ ★
CHILDREN: ★ ★ ★ ★
DIFFICULTY: ★ ★
SOLITUDE: ★ ★

THE CABIN IS THE CENTER OF MAPLE SUGAR PROCESSING EACH SPRING.

GPS TRAILHEAD COORDINATES: N39° 58.813' W82° 24.818'

DISTANCE & CONFIGURATION: 2.7-mile loop

HIKING TIME: About 2 hours

HIGHLIGHTS: Plant collections, gardens, ponds

ELEVATION: 990' at trailhead; 910' to 1,036' overall

ACCESS: Daily, 7 a.m.–sunset; no fees or permits required

MAPS: At visitor center (open Monday–Saturday, 8 a.m.–5 p.m.; Sunday, 10 a.m.–5 p.m.); **dawesarb.org**

FACILITIES: Visitor center, gift shop, nature center, drinking water, restrooms

WHEELCHAIR ACCESS: Yes; 4.5-mile auto tour

COMMENTS: Pets must be leashed; collecting of plant material not permitted

CONTACTS: 7770 Jacksontown Rd. SE, Newark, OH 43056; 800-443-2937; **dawesarb.org**

Overview

The Oak Trail is the longest hiking trail at Dawes Arboretum, which gives hikers the most interaction with this special place. The numerous collections of trees and plants are grouped in sections, and the Oak Trail finds its way through nearly every assembly. With all the beautiful displays, the hike is over before you know it. A short companion loop will have you walking on stones a few inches above the pond surface in the Japanese Garden. Near the end of the Dawes adventure, hikers enter a deep wood and take a boardwalk stroll through a cypress swamp, which will keep the camera shutter clicking.

Route Details

After watching the working beehive at the nature center, slip the pack on your back and head out the front door to the stone-paved patio a few steps to the west. From there, begin the Oak Trail, marked with signposts etched with a white oak leaf. The well-maintained gravel path heads west, and a few yards into the hike, a mature white oak tree stands guard over the route just as it bursts out into the open. Winding down a gentle hillside, the trail passes an agricultural display in mini form; check out the windmill, corn plantings, sunflower plot,

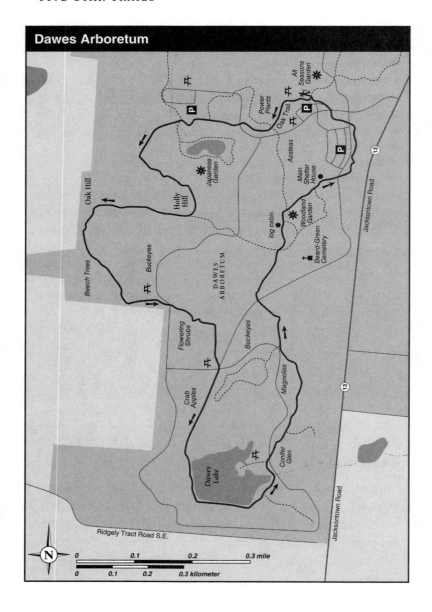

Dawes Arboretum

and split rail fencing. At 0.2 mile the Maple Trail intersects from the south and joins the Oak Trail.

Next you'll cross a park road, and then 400 feet ahead on the left you'll find the Japanese Garden access trail—a worthy side trip that balloons and returns here. The Oak Trail transitions from gravel to grass, but it's easy to identify as it continues west through a meadow. The path curves to the south and arrives at the base of a hill covered with mature deciduous trees. An interpretive sign offers details on the ecosystem where meadow and woodland meet. Up through the woods you go. It's not steep, but it will get your heart pumping as you climb. Halfway up the hill, a trail slips off to the left. It's not marked, but our Oak Trail bears to the right and soon arrives on Holly Hill—home to a collection of holly plants. At the top, a small sitting shelter splits the Oak and Holly Trails that have shared the same path from the visitor center—the Holly Trail goes left (east), but you turn right (west) to stay on the Oak Trail. Nearly each plant and tree has an identification tag. Keep an eye out for the deciduous holly tree on the left of the trail soon after departing the shelter.

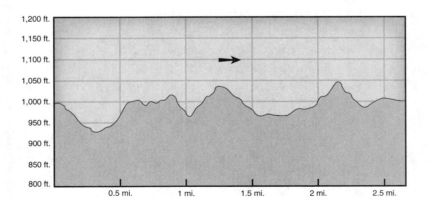

Continuing west on the ridge, the trail leaves the hollies and begins a curve. At 0.8 mile into the hike you're sitting on top of Oak Hill. Oaks both big and small decorate the peak. Look to the northwest to get a glimpse of the village of Heath. On the south slope, the beech and buckeye collections are the next native residents on display. These trees are not in a forest setting, but instead, decorate mowed landscapes. The trail continues on a meadow path, turning east at the hill base. The trail crosses the park road again at 1.1 miles.

Working your way uphill through a collection of mixed shrubs, short trees, and a stately row of maples on the left, the trail turns south again. At 1.3 miles the trail crosses through a parking loop where some auto tour explorers stop for a quick stroll. A billboard with map and event information sits near the road here. Cross the park road and enter the tree-lined, grassy lane known as Pershing Avenue, featuring tree species commonly planted along town streets. Many bear plaques in honor of America's military veterans. The 10-yard-wide path is a pleasant stretch to walk, especially in the fall when the foliage bursts with color. Dawes Lake appears on the left as you travel south on Pershing, so take a left and saunter along the lake's three-sided dam. While standing on the dam's most southerly point, gander at the interestingly shaped rows and curves of arborvitae shrubs, a type of cedar, at the base of the dam. From the air, or from the observation tower rising above the southeast corner of the arboretum property, the grouping spells "Dawes Arboretum."

The trail turns north after reaching the east side of the lake. On the right, at 1.7 miles, a spur trail leads to the observation tower. Back on the Oak Trail, 500 feet ahead, a wheelchair-accessible spur trail on the left leads out to a small island. A few steps north of that spur, Oak Trail crosses the park road and enters the Conifer Glen and then into meadow with magnolias before reaching the edge of the Deep Woods. That stretch from the lake island spur to the Deep Woods is 0.25 mile. A spur trail to the left here leads to the Rare Tree Collection.

The Deep Woods is a mature forest with a healthy ecosystem of thick saplings, towering deciduous trees, and decaying logs. The trail crosses the park road again at the peak of the hill and remains on a north track through the forest. At 2.25 miles the Holly Trail joins from the west. And 200 feet downhill is the path to the log cabin, a maple syrup station in the spring. The Maple Trail turns left from the Oak Trail 100 feet ahead. At 2.5 miles the path again crosses the park road and enters the Cypress Swamp on a boardwalk. The trail parallels the park road for 400 feet and then arrives at the main parking area at the visitor center.

Nearby Attractions

Drive 4.25 miles north on OH 13 to Hopewell Drive. Follow Hopewell Drive for 2 miles to OH 79. Turn right on OH 79 and then make an immediate left into the Great Circle Earthworks—a National Historic Landmark. The circular mound was built by the Hopewell Indians nearly 2,000 years ago. As the museum reveals, the mounds are believed to be astronomical observatories for the native culture. Also on site is the Licking County Visitors Bureau. South on OH 79 is a row of restaurants and retail stores.

Directions

From Columbus, take I-70 east for 32.37 miles to Exit 132. Follow OH 13 north for 2.6 miles to the arboretum entrance on the left.

Denison University Biological Reserve

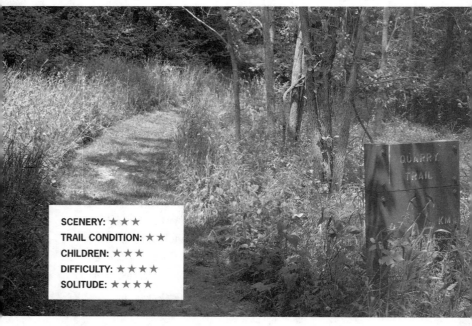

SCENERY: ★ ★ ★
TRAIL CONDITION: ★ ★
CHILDREN: ★ ★ ★
DIFFICULTY: ★ ★ ★ ★
SOLITUDE: ★ ★ ★ ★

THE QUARRY TRAIL IS ONE OF SEVERAL SIDE TRAILS AT THE RESERVE.

GPS TRAILHEAD COORDINATES: N40° 05.026' W82° 31.209'

DISTANCE & CONFIGURATION: 4.4-mile loop

HIKING TIME: About 3.5 hours

HIGHLIGHTS: Ponds, deep forest, solitude

ELEVATION: 1,043' at trailhead; 887' to 1,126' overall

ACCESS: Daily, sunrise–sunset

MAPS: At trailhead and **tinyurl.com/dureserve**

FACILITIES: None

WHEELCHAIR ACCESS: No

COMMENTS: Firearms, campfires, camping, and disturbance of natural features are prohibited.

CONTACTS: 740-587-0810; **franksb@denison.edu; tinyurl.com/dureserve**

Overview

Explore a wide valley floor and its meadows, tree rows, and ponds flourishing with wildlife. Stay on the trails, as you will see many red flags marking various research plantings. Enjoy the forest of mixed hardwoods before arriving at a stand of mature conifers. Travel up and over a series of ravines covered with a forest canopy interrupted by a few brushy runs on sunny open sections.

Route Details

Natural area and ecosystem research thrives north of Granville at the 350-acre Denison University Biological Reserve. This largely forested area is within walking distance of the college, but it doesn't get as many visitors as you might think. According to Denison, the purpose of the reserve is "to enhance the education of students in Biology and the Environmental Sciences." The reserve is open to the public, allowing us to reap the benefits of the university's scholarly research. The reserve consists of three contiguous land sections connected by a series of 15 hiking trails. The outing detailed here uses eight of those trails, touching on all of the reserve's habitats.

We begin at the small parking area at the Polly Anderson Field Station (home to the on-site laboratory). A bulletin board provides trail alerts, if any, and outlines reserve regulations. Down the slope from the bulletin board is the map box and trailhead identification sign. The trail system is a bit complicated, but it's understandable if you study the map for a few minutes before embarking on your hike. The Whitetail Loop trail is the first to invite you into the reserve. It's a mix of gravel and grass but wide enough for a couple to walk side by side—not all of the trails here are as well groomed, so be sure your boots (and feet) are ready for a workout.

Although the maze of trails may cause you to stop and recheck your map often, the trailheads are well marked with painted wood signs. If you have a handheld GPS unit, this may be a fun place to gain some practice with it for more advanced treks in the future. The first

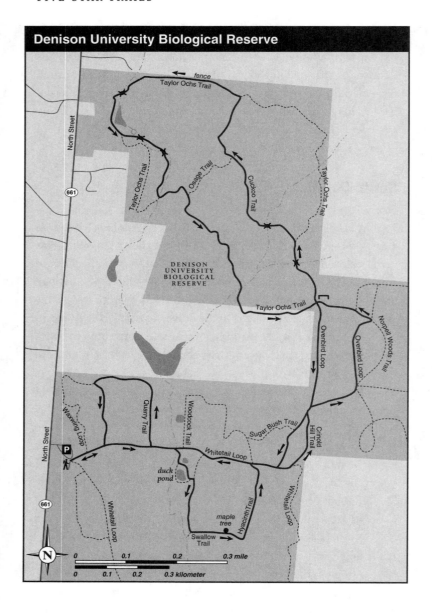

Denison University Biological Reserve

trail to connect to the Whitetail Loop is the Waxwing Loop, which joins from the north. It's a short loop that provides a view of the field station and surrounding grounds. Just 300 feet from the parking area is the second add-on path, the Quarry Trail. We'll follow that one on the way back. At 0.25 mile from the trailhead a pond lurks behind some brushy tree cover on the right. A mowed area offers a link to the Whitetail Loop and the pond, and a second pond a few yards to the south; both ponds are accessible from surrounding pathways. The ponds' residents include turtles, frogs, and sun-loving snakes, which use the occasional log left in the pond for habitat.

After a few steps farther on the Whitetail Loop, you'll see the Swallow Trail head off to the right—take that. It follows the perimeter of a field, where a few rows of bird boxes stand atop 6-foot steel posts. When the field's vegetation reaches knee-high, and insects are plentiful and buzzing about, swallows by the dozens come to feed all afternoon—an impressive air show to enjoy. The Swallow Trail soon passes by a tree-lined creek, then a grove of hardwoods on the right, and finally a stand of young spruces and flowering trees on the left, providing more wildlife observation possibilities. The trail then runs into the Hyacinth Trail at the

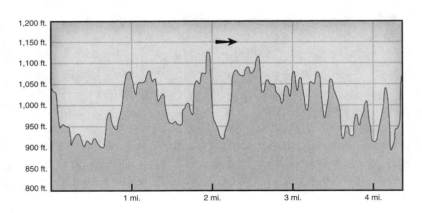

0.7-mile mark—take a left and follow the Hyacinth Trail north to rejoin the Whitetail Loop.

Back on the Whitetail Loop, go right (east) and into the woods to find the Crinoid Hill Trail, bypassing the Woodcock and Sugar Bush Trails on the way. The Whitetail Loop carries on to the east and makes a large loop back to the parking area, but you turn north on the Crinoid Hill Trail and travel 0.1 mile up a steep, narrow dirt trail (watch for sprawling tree roots) to the intersection of the Ovenbird, Sugar Bush, and Crinoid Trails. After catching your breath from the climb, stay to the right and follow the Ovenbird Trail's northeasterly option—you will be returning on the western leg of the same trail. As you cross the ridge, a stand of mature Norway spruce and white pines offers a pleasing aroma similar to a western state's conifer forest. The Norpell Woods Trail touches the Ovenbird path twice before the latter trail finds the Taylor Ochs Trail at 1.3 miles.

The Taylor Ochs Trail completes a loop around the remote northern block of the reserve, while the Cuckoo Trail cuts through the center (north/south) of the block. Follow the Taylor Ochs Trail to the north 0.2 mile, then turn left on the Cuckoo Trail. The Cuckoo travels through a typical central Ohio hardwood forest, with patches of brush squeezing in against the trail occasionally for about 0.5 mile, and crosses one valley and a creek. At the reserve's northern border, the Cuckoo Trail meets the circling Taylor Ochs Trail—turn left and follow Taylor Ochs. At 2.25 miles, the trail passes a small woodland pond that displays several research projects in progress. Don't touch any objects along the pond edge, but you're free to wonder what the students are learning here.

From the research pond, hike 0.75 mile up and over a hardwood-forested ridge and return to the Ovenbird Trail. At the intersection of the Ovenbird and Taylor Ochs Trails, where you began the Taylor Ochs section, follow the Ovenbird down the hill and across a pretty wooded valley. At 3.5 miles the Sugar Bush Trail veers off to the right. Follow it down to the Whitetail Loop (where you came in) and hike west 0.3 mile back to the 0.4-mile Quarry Trail. This hike will test your orienteering skills. If you get lost, don't worry. One of the students checking in on the research projects will find you before you starve.

Nearby Attractions

The village of Granville, home of Denison University, offers a quiet downtown with cafés, restaurants, and shops to explore. The main thoroughfare, East Broadway, rolls out the red carpet for visitors, with a wide sidewalk patio for dining and conversation. Moundbuilders State Memorial is 6 miles to the southeast in Newark. The museum reveals hundreds of amazing facts about the Hopewell culture that thrived here more than 2,000 years ago.

Directions

From Columbus, travel east on OH 16 for 24 miles to Granville. Turn right (east) on Broadway for 0.3 mile to OH 661. Follow OH 661 north for 1.25 miles to the reserve entrance on the right.

17 # Flint Ridge
State Memorial

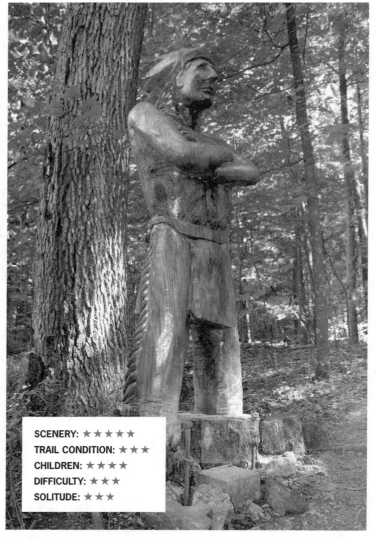

SCENERY: ★ ★ ★ ★ ★
TRAIL CONDITION: ★ ★ ★
CHILDREN: ★ ★ ★ ★
DIFFICULTY: ★ ★ ★
SOLITUDE: ★ ★ ★

THE AMERICAN INDIAN HISTORY AT THIS PARK IS DEEP AND EVIDENT STILL.

GPS TRAILHEAD COORDINATES: N39° 59.239' W82° 15.737'

DISTANCE & CONFIGURATION: 2.7-mile loop

HIKING TIME: About 2 hours

HIGHLIGHTS: Woodlands, American Indian flint mining pits

ELEVATION: 1,173' at trailhead; 1,249' at highest point

ACCESS: Daily, sunrise–sunset; no fees or permits required

MAPS: At the park museum and trailhead bulletin board

FACILITIES: Restrooms, drinking fountain, picnic area, museum

WHEELCHAIR ACCESS: Yes, restrooms and 0.25-mile paved trail with Braille interpretive signs

COMMENTS: Pets must be leashed; no bikes; gathering flint prohibited.

CONTACTS: 3800 Pleasant Chapel Road SE, Newark, OH 43056; 800-283-8707; ohiohistory.org/flintridge

Overview

The American Indians considered this wide ridge an important source of the vital mineral flint. Today, the material and the efforts to extract it remain the highlight of the place. Trails lead trekkers through the maze of ancient flint quarries and the surrounding deciduous forest that covers the ridge and its slopes. Allow extra time to pause and reflect on the edge of the shallow quarries and ponder the lives lived here hundreds of years ago.

Route Details

Flint Ridge State Memorial (FRSM) is a jewel in the Ohio Historical Society's crown. The abundance of access at the park allows visitors to get a deep look at the park's theme and history. Three trails of varying length welcome all levels of physical abilities; all trails leave from and return to the paved walkway that leads from the parking area to the museum. The museum is open weekends May through October; the trails are open year-round.

Starting at the park's entrance, a wide, level lawn the size of a football field spreads out on the left. This is the picnic area, which includes modern restrooms and a shelter house. Going past

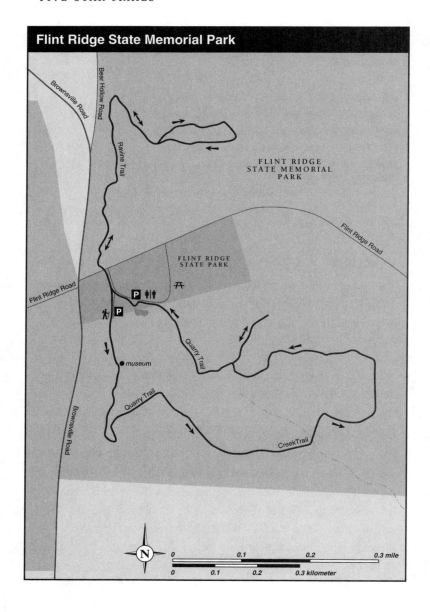

Flint Ridge State Memorial Park

FLINT RIDGE
STATE MEMORIAL
PARK

FLINT RIDGE
STATE PARK

Brownsville Road

Bear Hollow Road

Ravine Trail

Flint Ridge Road

Flint Ridge Road

Brownsville Road

Quarry Trail

Quarry Trail

CreekTrail

museum

N

0   0.1   0.2   0.3 mile

0   0.1   0.2   0.3 kilometer

the paved lane that turns to the shelter house, the parking area for the museum and trail is straight ahead. After parking, look for a paved trail heading south to the museum, which is tucked into the forest edge. The museum's abundant displays and extensive artifact collection can soak up an hour or more, so if possible, plan your visit during a day that the museum is open ($3 fee). If you visit first, the walk among the flint pits will mean much more.

From the museum, turn south toward a map sign and a wooden statue of an American Indian, flanking both sides of the gravel/dirt path. This is the Quarry Trail, marked with blue blazes. At 0.1 mile along the Quarry Trail, the Wagon Road Shortcut takes off to the left and reconnects to the Quarry Trail later in the hike. Stay on the Quarry Trail, following it to Deep Flint Pit—one of the largest on the property. A mix of hardwood trees provides a cooling canopy over the deeper pits. The Quarry Trail continues between numerous flint pits, before turning left and east, and then north toward the rear of the museum. At 0.25 mile the Wagon Road Shortcut returns to the main path. The trail continues to wind slightly through the deciduous forest, passing shallow, 5-yard-wide flint pits. Walking among the pits is like crossing a bombarded crater field. You'll

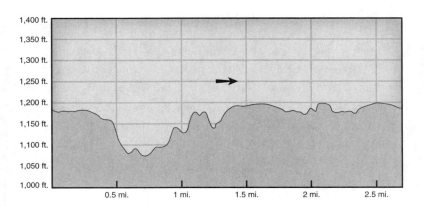

definitely want to plan extra time for this section, as the pits are attention-absorbing. At 0.3 mile take the 1-mile Creek Trail (marked with wooden sign) to the right (east). The Quarry Trail continues north, and before reaching the picnic area, the Creek Trail will rejoin it. If the pits have consumed more time than you had planned, skip the Creek Trail and stay on the Quarry Trail to get back on schedule.

If you take the Creek Trail, after just a few steps, you'll see the amount of flint fragments increases. The majority of these colorful pieces are from the flint formation that lies just beneath the soil here. Some of the pieces also may have been discarded by the American Indians. Each Labor Day, the Flint Ridge Knap-In is held at the picnic area. Hundreds of flint knappers demonstrate the skills and techniques used by the American Indians to create hunting and other tools from flint. Large flint chunks are stacked into a 3-foot-high pile near the base of a huge oak tree on the left side of the trail as it begins to leave the ridge and descend into a wide hollow.

The forest covering the hollow offers an impressive show of vibrant colors during autumn. The orange and red leaves temporarily cover the similarly colored flint on the forest floor. During springtime, the hollow's bottom is blanketed with a mix of wildflowers that attract butterflies. Pack your butterfly identification book. Beginning at the 0.6-mile mark, the first of four wooden bridges crosses one of a small network of trickling streams coursing through the bottom. The trail rounds back toward the museum and begins to climb the northern side of the hollow. The path has less flint on this stretch compared to the ridgetop, but flanking the forest are flint boulders available for inspection—watch your fingers, as the flint is sharp. At 1 mile, the Creek Trail is nearing the north intersection with the Quarry Trail, but before that, a spur trail on the right winds up the ridge to a flint outcropping. The trailhead is marked, but downed logs and little foot traffic makes the spur trail a bit challenging to follow anytime except summer.

At 1.3 miles the Creek Trail rejoins the Quarry Trail. Turn right and hike north, following the blue blazes to the picnic area. This concludes the primary hike. Grab a drink at the water fountain at the picnic area parking lot and follow the paved park road north to the park entrance and cross Flint Ridge Road for a bonus hike. This mowed trail is new and was not included on the map at press time. The Ravine Trail is a 1-mile out-and-back that also passes by flint pits for the first 0.3 mile. The heavily blazed trail then follows the edge of a forested deep ravine. A couple of benches are placed at the ravine's edge, inviting a quiet rest. When you return to the trail's beginning, your vehicle will be within sight across the road and straight ahead.

Nearby Attractions

The "Ridge," a privately owned museum located just west of the park on Flint Ridge Road, provides more insight to the history of the area. In the town of Heath, 12 miles to the northwest, you'll find the Great Circle Earthworks—a 1,200-foot circular mound used by the Hopewell culture for ceremonial events more than 2,000 years ago. A museum there describes additional American Indian sites to explore. To the northeast, follow OH 668 to Brushy Fork Road to find the west parking area for the Blackhand Nature Preserve and the popular paved 4-mile hike-and-bike trail that follows the Licking River, which is popular for canoeing throughout the summer.

Directions

From Columbus, take I-70 east 42 miles to Exit 141. Travel north on OH 668 for 0.9 mile to Brownsville. Turn left on US 40 and go 0.1 mile to OH 668 and turn right. Travel 3.1 miles north to Flint Ridge Road and turn right. The park entrance is the first lane on the right.

18

Hebron Fish Hatchery

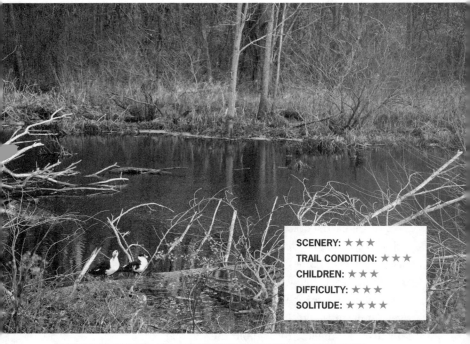

SCENERY: ★ ★ ★
TRAIL CONDITION: ★ ★ ★
CHILDREN: ★ ★ ★
DIFFICULTY: ★ ★ ★
SOLITUDE: ★ ★ ★ ★

THE HIDDEN SWAMPS AND PONDS ATTRACT THOUSANDS OF VARIOUS WATERFOWL SPECIES.

GPS TRAILHEAD COORDINATES: N39° 56.540' W82° 30.497'

DISTANCE & CONFIGURATION: 2.6-mile loop

HIKING TIME: About 2 hours

HIGHLIGHTS: Birdlife, wildlife, wetlands

ELEVATION: 879' at trailhead, with no significant rise

ACCESS: Closes at sunset; no fees or permits required

MAPS: At the park office on Canal Road and **tinyurl.com/hebronmap**

FACILITIES: Restrooms in Administration Building (Monday–Friday, 8 a.m.–3 p.m.)

WHEELCHAIR ACCESS: No

COMMENTS: During very wet periods, the trail can see some flooding in the middle and southern property sections.

CONTACTS: 10517 Canal Road, Hebron, OH 43025; 740-928-8092; **www2.ohiodnr.com**

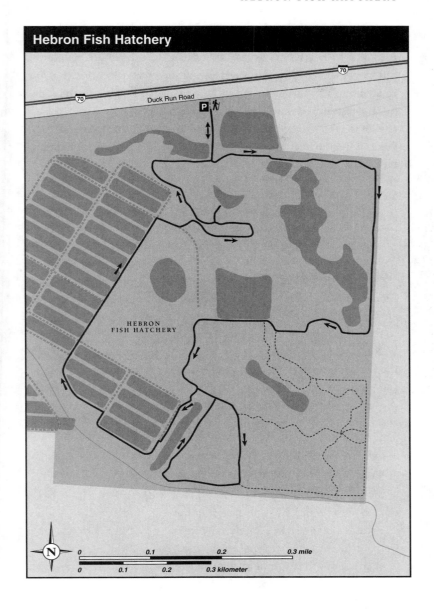

Overview

Although hatcheries are usually about fish, it's the birdlife here that attracts hikers. The 25-acre wetland will hold your attention as you tread along and through the carefully managed swamp. In the fall, multiple species of waterfowl pause there to rest in mid-migration to the south. You should pause yourself to listen and watch for flocks of ducks lining up a landing or taking off. Green herons and the larger blue heron are regularly heard croaking overhead. A jaunt through the 50-acre wet woods will surround you with a variety of wildlife and birdlife calling to each other and offering photo ops galore. Pack extra camera batteries. The park was designated a Watchable Wildlife Area by the Ohio Division of Wildlife.

Route Details

From the trailhead on Duck Run Road, north of the main hatchery entrance, Interstate 70 and its traffic can be seen and heard 200 feet to the north, but once on the trail, it soon disappears. The trailhead parking is a small gravel area marked with a 6-foot sign identifying the hatchery property. Walk to the left of the sign and past a metal gate and the main trail heads straight south. Just 100 feet down the trail two large oak trees stand at the edge of a wetland pond. A brushy field to the west regularly radiates with birdsong provided by warblers and sparrows.

At 0.1 mile you'll reach a T in the road and a small, white sign pointing to four waterfowl hunting blinds (used on a few weekends in the fall). Turn left and follow the 30-foot-wide, mowed path to the east. Private property lies to the left of the trail, and a lively wetland entertains on the right. The dry rises that spread out through the wetland like earthen fingers are favored by the white-tailed deer population. If you're slow and quiet you'll have a chance of observing a majestic buck showing off his antlers.

The trail remains wide and well mowed throughout the hatchery's trail network, narrowing only through the woodlands. The path turns south and at 0.6 mile, sitting at the edge of a wetland pond, is Blind 4 (a small wooden shelter for waterfowl hunters, only accessible by wading). A couple hundred feet farther south, a wide trail turns to the right (west)—take that option. The trail soon narrows and follows the woods' edge to the southeast corner of the property. During rains, this portion of trail floods, so I suggest avoiding it. The westerly trail parallels a tall grass meadow off to the left. To the right, a short side trail takes off and curves through the wetland edge and then swings back to the main trail. At 0.75 mile the wide grass trail arrives at an intersection. Turning left leads back to the south-heading trail section and turning right brings you to a square pond—take that option. A few steps and you're already at the pond's edge.

Follow the mowed road west along the pond's southern bank toward a secluded equipment shed. A trail marked by an orange sign reading AREA 2 leads into the woods south of the shed—follow this trail. The trail bed is primarily gravel, offering a solid base as it enters the wet woods. One wild resident that's seldom seen is the endangered massasauga rattlesnake. This swamp-dwelling reptile prefers to soak up sunrays on hot, humid days by stretching out on logs and stumps near the water's edge—stay on the path. Travel 0.1 mile to a trail arcing to the east. A few yards around the bend, a short trail turns off to the right and leads up to the raised banks of the fish-rearing ponds. You will return to this point later and take that trail to the ponds, but for now, go straight ahead.

At the 1-mile point, another trail takes off to the right, but again, continue straight for now. After hiking another 200 feet, the trail turns to the right—follow it. At that same point, a narrower, weedy trail breaks off to the left. That path, Trail 2, intersects the heart of the "Big Woods" but has several points that remain wet enough to require tall, waterproof boots unless it has been dry for a couple of weeks. The better main trail that you remain on passes between the dense woods and an old field, now a young woodlot. A level, easy stroll of 0.1 mile delivers you to the south property line and a grassy lane paralleling it.

Turn right and head west for another 0.1 mile, then turn right again and head north. To the left of the trail is a pond with downed trees covered in moss and aqua weeds sprouting out over the brush-covered water's edge. This pond is favored by waterfowl in both spring and fall, primarily because of its remoteness.

Take the grassy trail by the water for 0.2 mile to return to the main trail you covered while passing the rearing ponds. Turn left, walk about 100 feet, and turn left again to reach the first rearing pond and an elevated view of the isolated pond you followed on the opposing bank. Continue following the perimeter of the rearing pond roads to the south and then northwest until you reach the set of ponds southeast of the hatchery buildings. Follow the road heading northeast between the ponds and the woods to the east for 0.25 mile. At the second to last rearing pond from the north, turn right and descend on the gravel lane that leads to a mowed trail on the left. Follow the mowed trail to Blinds 2 and 3. Blind 3 is on the east side of the wildlife habitat field planting. Return to the north rearing pond and look for a grassy trail to bypass a brushy hump and head east 400 feet to the trail you started on. Turn left to return to the parking area.

Nearby Attractions

In the town of Buckeye Lake is the Greater Buckeye Lake Historical Society Museum, located at 4729 Walnut Road (OH 79). Local history displays include artifacts from a popular amusement park from the early 1900s. Other exhibits include mastodon bones unearthed near the lake, along with information on the Ohio-Erie Canal, developed in the early 1800s. The museum is open Tuesday–Sunday, 1–4 p.m. Across and down the street, is a favorite area restaurant, The Pizza Cottage.

Directions

From Columbus, take I-70 west for 25.8 miles to Exit 126. Follow OH 37 south 1 mile. Turn left on OH 79 and follow it east 1.4 miles. Turn left on Canal Road and travel 1 mile to the hatchery entrance, but pass the entrance and take the first right on Duck Run Road. Drive east 0.5 mile to a gravel parking area on the right.

19

Infirmary Mound Park

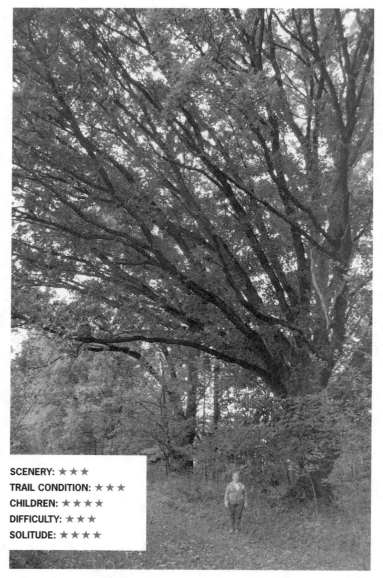

SCENERY: ★ ★ ★
TRAIL CONDITION: ★ ★ ★
CHILDREN: ★ ★ ★ ★
DIFFICULTY: ★ ★ ★
SOLITUDE: ★ ★ ★ ★

MATURE OAK TREES REMAIN STANDING TALL ALONG ABANDONED FENCE ROWS.

GPS TRAILHEAD COORDINATES: N40° 01.747' W82° 31.246'

DISTANCE & CONFIGURATION: 4-mile loop

HIKING TIME: About 3 hours

HIGHLIGHTS: Wildflowers, prairie, wildlife

ELEVATION: 1,039' at trailhead; 812' to 1,063' overall

ACCESS: Closes at sunset; no fees or permits required

MAPS: Print from **lickingparkdistrict.com**

FACILITIES: Shelter houses, portable toilets, drinking water

WHEELCHAIR ACCESS: No

COMMENTS: The trail is shared with equestrians.

CONTACTS: 740-587-2535; **lickingparkdistrict.com**

Overview

The trail travels over diverse topography, including prairie lands, steep hillsides, and mixed forest. Each turn exposes a change in wildlife habitat, which creates equally diverse viewing opportunities. Some trail sections are popular among equestrians, so watch your step. The hike starts at a lake's edge, and near the last leg of the trek, you will snake your way down into and back out of a wooded ravine. The varied terrain will keep your hiking boots limber.

Route Details

The Licking County Park District and its volunteers work hard to preserve wild places within a few miles of the suburbs. Hikers and nature lovers benefit from these labors. Infirmary Mound Park pleases all of the senses, and hiking here is just plain fun. From the only entrance to the park, follow the paved road straight to shelter house 6, which sets on the west shore of Mirror Lake (fishing permitted). Along the well-defined trail system, you'll find brown marking posts with numbers matching numbered points on the map—mostly at trail intersections or notable turns.

Walking north from shelter house 6, signpost 12 is near the lake's edge; continue 0.1 mile to signpost 11. A spur trail veers off

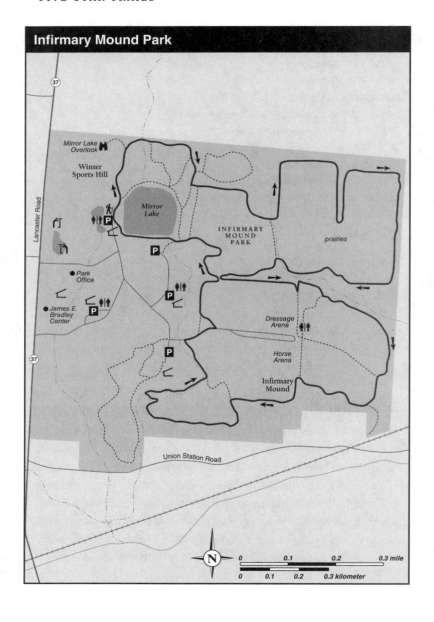

Infirmary Mound Park

to the left and up to the top of a mowed knoll called Mirror Lake Overlook. This is the northwest corner of the square-shaped, 326-acre park. The trail turns east at signpost 11 and narrows into a mix of saplings and brush. Because of the partial shade the grassy trail becomes dimpled during rains from horse feet, but it's not a big problem. Watch for white-tailed deer wandering from feeding to bedding areas. At 0.3 mile signpost 9 indicates a narrow side trail leading off to a wetland area on the right adjoining Mirror Lake. Our hike skips that option, staying on the primary trail, and soon arrives at signpost 8. On the left side of the path is the Wildflower Trail (no horses allowed), which makes a short loop through a tight, young forest.

From signpost 8, continue south for 0.03 mile to signpost 7 and turn left before pausing to photograph the lake from a slightly elevated viewpoint to the west. Enter the woods and immediately locate signpost 6—turn left and follow the dirt trail to signpost 5. You'll soon notice the contrast of young and old forest flanking both sides of the trail; old on the left and young on the right. During spring, you'll want to pause at this point for an entertaining show provided by songbirds. Turn left (north) at signpost 5. Bird nesting boxes are sporadically placed on trees along the left until the next turn. The trail's center shows signs of horse traffic as the path ascends to the north. At 0.75 mile four fields are grouped to the east and south. The trail follows the outside perimeter of the prairie that is divided into four sections by old fence rows crowded with trees and honeysuckle.

Heading east along the northern property border again, at 0.8 mile is a row of huge oak trees, one with a canopy more than 20 yards wide. The trail swings south, goes to the end of the tree row dividing the two northern fields, and then heads back north on the opposite side of the divider. The trail continues to follow the prairie's perimeter for 0.75 mile before reaching signpost 4 at the southwest corner of the prairie group. During late summer and early fall, the prairie grasses and intermingled brush hold an abundance of wildlife and dozens of butterfly species. Signpost 4 sits on the edge of the wood line—once you reach it, turn left and go 0.1 mile to signpost 3. Turn left and take a few steps to signpost 15, then turn left again and walk east to the corner of the open field. Once at the corner, turn left into the forest and follow the narrow and lumpy dirt trail to signpost 17 at the edge of a well-managed hay field.

Continue on the trail as it reenters the woods heading southeast. The path descends to a drainage crossing, the most remote point in the park, and then emerges from the forest with an 80-yard-long meadow, with signpost 18 to the right. Hike south 0.1 mile along the meadow and forest edge to a T in the path; turn right. The trail remains narrow and climbs steeply through a brushy forest before arriving at the southern end of the hay field. The jaunt up the rugged hillside requires some cardio. Walk to the old barn in the hay field and look west to signpost 19. The horse arena sits 100 yards north of post 19; turn left and follow the field's edge south and then west. At 2.9 miles you will arrive at signpost 20 just inside the woods. Turn and look back east across the field to signpost 19. The American Indian mound that gives the park its name is visible in the field, down slope from the horse arena.

Turn left at signpost 20 and you'll soon be immersed in a dense young-old forest mix with several young trees leaning over the narrow dirt trail, creating a woody tunnel. For the next 0.3 mile the trail is only a couple of feet wide and trenched. The views of a wooded ravine are the prize for the effort, but watch your step. The trail snakes down through the gully, crossing a creek (no bridge), and meets signpost 21. Turn north, and signpost 22 is just ahead near a paved park road. Follow the road to the right for 100 feet to signpost 23 on the left; from there, 0.5 mile of easy hiking is all that remains. You'll return to signposts 15 and 3. At post 3, go left (west) and follow the flat trail through a woodlot to signpost 2; go left to signpost 1, a few yards to the west. Walk to the top of the lake dam and look to the west to see your ride home.

Nearby Attractions

Granville lies 2 miles to the north of the park. The town is home to Denison University, and dozens of charming businesses line the downtown streets. Various restaurants, from ice cream parlors to coffee shops, will refuel bushed hikers. Umbrella-covered patio tables are the norm, spread out on the city's wide sidewalks. Buckeye Lake, Ohio's oldest state park, is 7 miles south. The lake was built in 1826 to feed Ohio's early canal system. Nine boat-launch ramps and three public swimming areas provide plenty of access to this shallow 3,100-acre lake.

Directions

From Columbus, take I-70 east 25.2 miles to Exit 126. Travel north on OH 37 for 6.2 miles to the park entrance on the right.

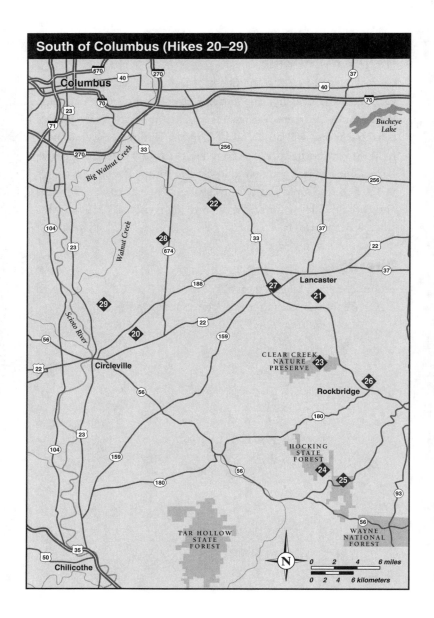

Columbus

Big Walnut Creek

Walnut Creek

Buckeye Lake

Lancaster

CLEAR CREEK NATURE PRESERVE

Rockbridge

Circleville

Scioto River

HOCKING STATE FOREST

TAR HOLLOW STATE FOREST

WAYNE NATIONAL FOREST

Chilicothe

0   2   4   6 miles

0   2   4   6 kilometers

South

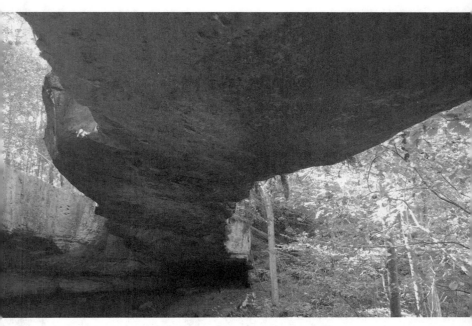

UNDER THE BRIDGE AT ROCKBRIDGE STATE NATURE PRESERVE.

20

A. W. Marion State Park

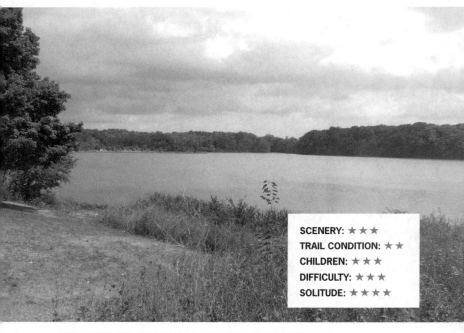

SCENERY: ★ ★ ★
TRAIL CONDITION: ★ ★
CHILDREN: ★ ★ ★
DIFFICULTY: ★ ★ ★
SOLITUDE: ★ ★ ★ ★

LAKE VIEWS ARE ABUNDANT ALONG THE HARGUS LAKE TRAIL.

GPS TRAILHEAD COORDINATES: N39° 37.987' W82° 53.057'

DISTANCE & CONFIGURATION: 3.8-mile loop

HIKING TIME: About 2 hours

HIGHLIGHTS: Lake views, woodlands

ELEVATION: 865' at trailhead, with no significant rise

ACCESS: Year-round, daily, sunrise–11 p.m.

MAPS: At concession store at boat rental and **tinyurl.com/awmarionmap**

FACILITIES: Latrines, drinking water, picnic areas, camping, pay phone

WHEELCHAIR ACCESS: No

COMMENTS: Pets must be leashed at all times. The hiking trail passes through the campground; please respect campers and remain quiet.

CONTACTS: 7317 Warner Huffer Road, Circleville, OH 43113; 740-869-3124; **tinyurl.com/awmarion**

Overview

A canoe gliding across the surface of Hargus Lake is only one of the pleasant scenes a hiker may encounter while circling the shore. Hargus Lake Trail runs through a hardwood forest, up and down ridges, and crosses ravines and tributaries feeding the pretty lake. Pause atop a lakeside bluff and gaze down at the water lightly licking the southern shoreline. The west side of the lakeshore is dotted with picnic areas and playgrounds, which are the only locations in this quiet little park that get busy.

Route Details

This park and its lake cover only 309 acres, but you'll have nearly 4 miles of opportunity for exploration, via the Hargus Lake Trail. Park maps and trail signs claim the hike is 5 miles. It's not, but nonetheless, the trail provides a diverse landscape, from lakeside walking to forested hill climbing to strolling through grassland. On arrival, the park's quiet atmosphere lures visitors to slow down and transition to a tranquil mood.

A trailhead sign stands near the boat ramp at the park entrance. Travel north on the Hargus Lake Trail, following the blue blazes. The beginning section is also used regularly by anglers fishing from shore, which is just a short walk from the paved parking area. Every dozen yards a dirt path jets over the bank edge to the water. If you packed a travel rod and reel, make a few casts before getting serious about your hike. Afterward, if you left your canoe or kayak at home, you can rent a rowboat from the concession store to further pursue a largemouth bass.

At a few points early on the trail mulch helps subdue the muddy sections. As the trail gets farther from the boat ramp and the fishing-access points, the path narrows and shows less sign of wear. The path passes around a narrow lake cove on the right and a camping resort on the left. Then it leads up into the woods, offering a glimpse of the lake through the trees. You'll encounter multiple sets

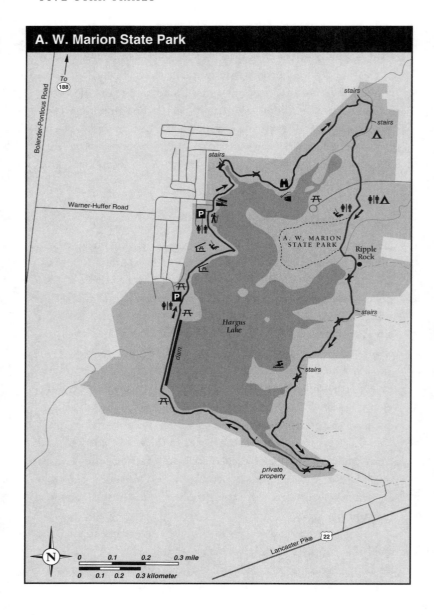

A. W. Marion State Park

of stairs on this trail; some are easily negotiable for the average adult, while others require some agility. The first set calls for high stepping, as the rises are more than 1 foot tall. Staying on course is not difficult for two reasons: the trail gets enough foot traffic to keep vegetation from hiding the path, and blue blazes are frequently placed on both standing trees and the occasional downfall.

The walk through the forest doesn't venture too far from the lake, although the water is now nearly out of sight. The trail begins to work its way back lakeside, descending a steep run from the hillside where the trail is studded with rocks for traction. You'll even find a few stairs on the steepest part. During dry weather, hikers cross Hargus Creek simply by walking on the creek bed; when water does flow ankle deep, stepping stones (and concrete blocks) allow for a dry crossing. After crossing the creek, up the hill you go on a flight of stairs, and then along the ridge to reach the campground at 1.2 miles. It sits on a ridge among large deciduous trees. Except for holiday weekends, the campground is lightly occupied. Enter the campground and walk straight to site 26. The Hargus Lake Trail passes to the right of the campsite; if it's occupied, be sure not to tread through the site, respecting the campers' privacy.

Signposts with blue blazes guide you through the campground and into the forest where the path will start to descend a razor ridge with an attractive ravine to the left. A second hiking trail, or nature trail as it is titled, leaves the campground at the same point as the Hargus Lake Trail. The Squawroot Trail does a 0.7-mile loop throughout a forested peninsula. However, you should continue on the Hargus Lake Trail, which bears to the left and continues south along the forested hills rolling down into the lake. Westerly breezes blow off the water and up into the forest—a pleasant relief from the heat in the summer and an added element to prepare for on winter hikes. Occasionally along the trail, you will come across a small, narrow spur leading toward the lake. Those were created by adventurous anglers getting away from the easy access points.

A set of stairs leads downhill at 1.7 miles. Some of the square wooden beams used in constructing the steps are missing, but the steel rebar stakes used to anchor them are still there—watch your step, as these little pegs stick up 6 inches or so and blend in with the rock and dirt of the trail surface. Cross a small tributary on a footbridge and climb up to traverse another ridge. The east leg of this trail stays in the woods, but at high vantage points, narrow views of the lake appear. Hike this trail in October for the best views of the lake and surrounding forest. Various birds, such as the downy woodpecker, visit the lakeside woods and also frequent the fields at the forest edge.

A bridge over a creek (at 2.4 miles) at the lake's most southern point gives hikers access to a pool of water for cooling the feet. At that same bridge, you may hear gunshots up the ravine, many gunshots actually. It's safe, though, as a monitored firearm range borders the park there. Follow the southern lakeshore for 0.2 mile beyond the creek crossing, then exit the tree cover and stroll through at the edge of a mowed lawn. Stay at the edge, following the blue blazes, as the yard to the left is private property. At 3 miles, the trail emerges into the open and passes across the gravel and sandy shoreline. Cross the dam heading north, and at the north end of the dam, follow the shoreline (blue blazes are sporadic for the last 0.5 mile) through picnic areas. Wide-angle views of the lake demand attention, so expect several stops for reflection on the way to your vehicle—or boat rental.

Nearby Attractions

Stage's Pond State Nature Preserve lies 6 miles to the north of A. W. Marion State Park. Stage's Pond offers hiking trails (detailed in this book on pages 192–197) that explore the waterfowl habitat of a kettle lake and the wildlife of a mixed forest. The city of Circleville, just west of the state park, hosts the annual Circleville Pumpkin Show in mid-October. The popular festival began in 1903. Today, it includes a parade, pumpkin judging, and hundreds of unique foods made with pumpkin.

Directions

From I-270 Exit 52, follow US 23 south 20 miles to Circleville and US 22 exit. Turn left at the end of the exit ramp and travel east on US 22 for 3 miles to Bolender-Pontious Road. Turn left and travel north 1.5 miles to Warner-Huffer Road. Turn right and drive 0.5 mile to the parking lot near the boat ramp.

Alley Park

SCENERY: ★ ★ ★ ★
TRAIL CONDITION: ★ ★ ★
CHILDREN: ★ ★ ★
DIFFICULTY: ★ ★ ★
SOLITUDE: ★ ★ ★ ★ ★

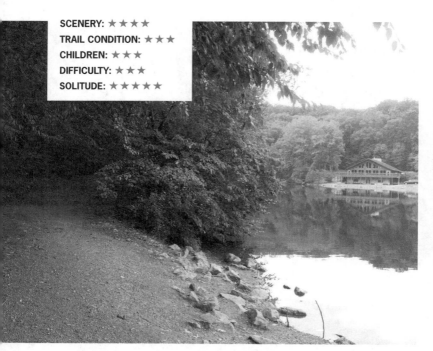

A PICTURESQUE SCENE OF THE PARK'S LODGE REFLECTED IN THE LAKE

GPS TRAILHEAD COORDINATES: N39° 40.789' W82° 34.787'

DISTANCE & CONFIGURATION: 1.5-mile loop

HIKING TIME: About 1.5 hours

HIGHLIGHTS: Remote forest lake, woodlands, covered bridge

ELEVATION: 890' at trailhead; 947' at highest point

ACCESS: Year-round, daily, sunrise–sunset

MAPS: Map board posted on bulletin board at park entrance and at **www.lancasterparks.com**

FACILITIES: Restroom, rental lodge, picnic area, nature center, drinking water

WHEELCHAIR ACCESS: Not on trails

COMMENTS: Pets must be kept on a leash. Catch-and-release fishing is permitted on two stocked lakes.

CONTACTS: 2805 Old Logan Road, Lancaster, OH 43130; 740-687-6651; **www.lancasterparks.com**

Overview

This 300-acre park is packed with a network of hiking trails covering it all. Our hike starts at the lodge overlooking the park's easily accessed fishing lake. A wide, groomed stone path sneaks out of the lodge parking lot and climbs a forested ridge. After reaching the top, it spills over the south side and arrives at a remote lake. Enjoy a waterside break, then travel around the ridge at a lower point to return to the main lake. Cross a dam, and then explore a smaller ridge viewpoint before returning down to the lodge parking area. This hike includes the Blackhand, Lakes, Twin Lakes, Alley, Buck Run, and Christmas Ferns Trails.

Route Details

While driving up the paved lane from the park entrance, a picturesque scene emerges between two ridges on the left. A pretty lake, with the reflection of the park's inviting lodge on the opposite shore, welcomes visitors. The lodge is available for parties and also serves as a nature center. A reconstructed log cabin and a covered bridge surrounded by picnic tables are other amenities at this pleasant park.

The lodge parking lot is used mainly by lodge guests, although hikers can park there if space allows. If the lodge and the paved parking lot are occupied, simply park in the area near the park entrance and trek up the lodge lane to begin the hike. Starting at the lodge parking lot, seek the Blackhand Trail, which appears to be a stone lane leading off into the forest at the southern edge of the parking lot. Trail options soon lead off to the right and then to the left. Nearly every intersection and connection is identified with small "You Are Here" maps attached to the top of short posts.

The Cove Trail offers a quick avenue to get a peek of the back bay of the lodge lake—Lake Loretta. Blackhand Trail turns to the east and begins to ascend a steep ridge. Even though the Blackhand Trail is tractor-wide, the tree canopy keeps it shaded. The farther the

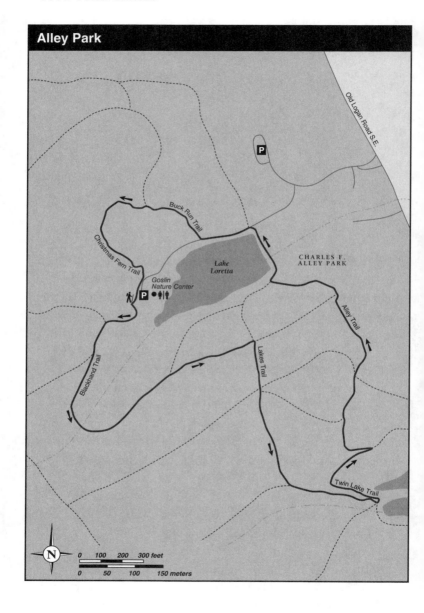

Alley Park

Old Logan Road S.E.

Buck Run Trail

Christmas Fern Trail

Lake
Loretta

CHARLES F.
ALLEY PARK

Goslin
Nature Center

Blackhand Trail

Lakes Trail

Alley Trail

Twin Lake Trail

N

| 0 | 100 | 200 | 300 feet |
| 0 | 50 | 100 | 150 meters |

trails extend into the remote parts of the park, the narrower they become due to less foot traffic and a diminished need for heavier trail maintenance. At 0.3 mile the Muskrat Bend Trail slips off downhill and follows Lake Loretta's southern edge across the dam to the paved park road—continue on the Blackhand Trail. The next trail to intersect the Blackhand Trail is the Lakes Trail. At that intersection, turn right for a jaunt up to the ridgetop, where you'll arrive at another trail intersection. This intersecting trail is aptly named Ridge Trail. Cross Ridge Trail (at the 0.5-mile point) and continue on Lakes Trail for 0.2 mile to reach the Twin Lake Trail. On the way, you will pass Poplar Valley Trail on the right as the Lakes Trail runs down from the ridge.

At the junction of the Lakes and Twin Lake Trails, go straight to follow the Twin Lake Trail to a short, wooded peninsula jutting out into Twin Lake. During summer, the lake is covered with lily pads, and in spring listen for singing frogs. Twin Lake Trail surrounds the woodland lake, with several paths leading off from the roundabout trail. Plan to enjoy a break while sitting on a log and watching critters surface from the lake and crawl or slither

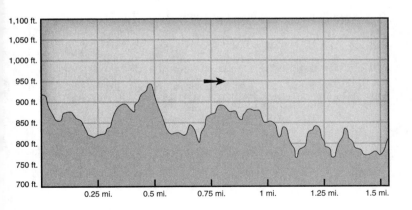

onto deadfall extending into the water. A camera zoom lens offers a sure way to get a close-up look. You may have the place to yourself because of the steep ridge standing between Twin Lake and the main park area.

Leave the peninsula and return to the Lakes–Twin Lake Trails junction. Travel north on Twin Lake Trail 0.1 mile to Alley Trail, which makes a sharp left turn. The Alley Trail is a 2.25-mile route that loops around the park, staying close to the park's boundaries. As our hike joins the Alley Trail from the Twin Lake Trail, the Alley Trail traverses around the downslope of the tall ridge you crossed while following the Lakes Trail. At 1 mile the Alley Trail touches the Ridge Trail on the left—bear right to stay on Alley Trail. A few yards past that point, the trail begins to descend the ridge. The path narrows due to less tree canopy, which creates more underbrush to crowd the trail; in a few spots the underbrush even provides a green curtain. A metal farm gate on the right at 1.1 miles marks the end of a park service road. At that point, Blackhand Trail joins from the left. Stay on the Alley Trail to arrive at Lake Loretta's dam.

Cross the dam slowly and give the lodge and lake another look—it's a beautiful setting. Waterfowl are frequent lake visitors, as are common water snakes, which offer additional targets for your zoomy camera. At 1.2 miles you will arrive at the paved park road that you drove in on. Follow it toward the lodge and take the next trail—Buck Run Trail—on the right. Buck Run will raise your heart rate by ramping uphill right from the start. As the trail begins to level off a bit, Christmas Fern Trail takes off to the left. Take it back down the fern-decorated ridge to arrive at the lodge parking lot.

Nearby Attractions

Fairfield County is considered the northern gateway to the Hocking Hills Region, which has several parks with geologic wonders accessible by miles of hiking trails. A couple of miles north of Alley Park is the pleasant town of Lancaster. For a list of historical sites and outdoor adventure opportunities, contact the Fairfield County Visitors and Convention Bureau at 800-626-1296, or check out **visitfairfieldcountyoh.org**

Directions

From Columbus, follow US 33 south 27 miles to the Tarkiln Road Exit. At the stop sign, turn left and go east 0.2 mile to Old Logan Road. Turn left and drive 1.5 miles to the park entrance on the left.

Chestnut Ridge Metro Park

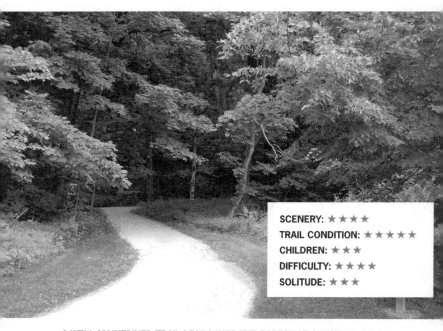

SCENERY: ★ ★ ★ ★
TRAIL CONDITION: ★ ★ ★ ★ ★
CHILDREN: ★ ★ ★
DIFFICULTY: ★ ★ ★ ★
SOLITUDE: ★ ★ ★

A WELL-MAINTAINED TRAIL LEADS INTO THE FOREST AT CHESTNUT RIDGE.

GPS TRAILHEAD COORDINATES: N39° 48.391' W82° 45.362'

DISTANCE & CONFIGURATION: 1.9-mile loop

HIKING TIME: About 1.5 hours

HIGHLIGHTS: Ridgetop views, meadows, forest environment, wildlife observation

ELEVATION: 882' at trailhead; 907' to 1,079' overall

ACCESS: Daily, 6:30 a.m.–sunset

MAPS: At bulletin boards in parking areas, ranger station, and **tinyurl.com/chestnutridgepark**

FACILITIES: Vault restrooms, drinking water fountains, picnic areas

WHEELCHAIR ACCESS: No

COMMENTS: Walking to top of ridge is a constant climb. For a less demanding trip, reverse route.

CONTACTS: 8445 Winchester Road NW, Carroll, OH 43112; 614-891-0700; **tinyurl.com/chestnutridgepark**

Overview

The Ridge Trail is all uphill for the first quarter of this hike. The climb through forested ridge is invigorating, but also informative thanks to several interpretive signs strategically placed along the trail. Once at the ridgetop, you'll find two observation decks, the first offering a view of the Columbus skyline. Drop to a lower elevation on the Meadows Trail to cross a creek meandering through a mixed grass meadow.

Route Details

The ridge that delivers a stimulating hike today still holds remnants of its past. A few decaying logs lying about the forest are more than 200 years old. The American chestnut trees that blanketed the ridge and gave it its name were wiped out by a blight during the early 1900s. An interpretive sign located on the east side of the Ridge Trail offers some details about the plight of the blight. You'll find remains of an orchard throughout the entire metro park. In the center of the trail loop, you'll find the foundation of the last farmhouse that called the ridge home. The meadow to the south of the old homestead may be devoid of crops, but it thrives now with birdlife and wildlife roaming the grassland and aquatic life wiggling wildly up and down the stream.

After entering the park's main entrance, bypass the ranger station and wetlands overlook on the left and turn right into the first parking area. Latrines, drinking water, and a picnic area with grills flank both sides of the parking area. The forest rises in front of you, and to the west you'll see the ridge you're there to explore. The crushed limestone, 8-foot-wide trail leads straight into the woods, passing a NO PETS ALLOWED ON TRAIL sign. Just into the woods, you'll be greeted by a sign announcing that this is indeed a hiking trail. Go right and begin the climb. There is much to see, hear, smell, and feel as you travel up the forest ridge—trees both old and young, owls, songbirds, woodpeckers, a forest carpet of leaves and vegetation, and the fresh air you will be sucking in. This stretch of the hike is memorable.

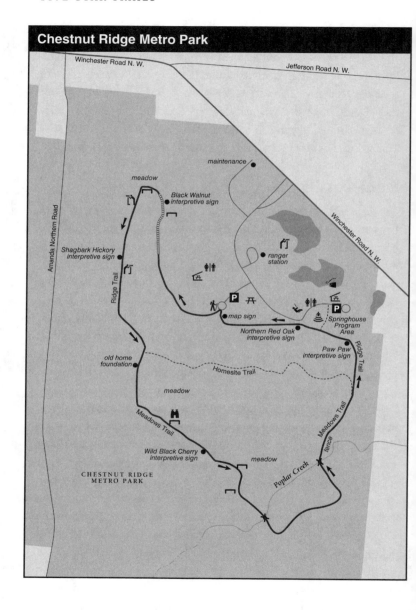

Chestnut Ridge Metro Park

Winchester Road N. W.

Jefferson Road N. W.

Amanda Northern Road

Winchester Road N. W.

maintenance

meadow

Black Walnut
interpretive sign

Shagbark Hickory
interpretive sign

Ridge Trail

ranger
station

map sign

Northern Red Oak
interpretive sign

P

Springhouse
Program
Area

Paw Paw
interpretive sign

old home
foundation

Homesite Trail

Ridge Trail

meadow

Meadows Trail

Meadows Trail

Wild Black Cherry
interpretive sign

meadow

Poplar Creek

fence

CHESTNUT RIDGE
METRO PARK

A quarter mile up, the trail surface turns to wood. Yes, wood. The ridge gets steeper to the left and right, so a boardwalk was constructed to level the trail side to side. The well-built walkway includes a strip of asphalt material for traction when wet, and a sturdy handrail keeps hikers from falling off the edge. The boardwalk runs along the east side of the ridge for 0.1 mile. The trail returns to stone surface and the incline increases for 100 feet or so before leveling off with a small field on the right and a bench on the left, a perfect site for wildlife photography. The trail turns south but continues climbing, and at 0.5 mile the observation deck appears on the right. The overlook has a few seats, and if the sky is not too hazy you can view the Columbus skyline on the horizon. Trees surround the deck except for the opening to the west.

Up the trail 0.1 mile from the first observation deck is a second deck. This one doesn't have a skyline view, but instead features a view of the forest below, along with an interpretive sign recounting a local author's experience on the ridge in the 1970s. After finally reaching the peak of the ridge at the 0.75-mile mark, you'll see a piece or two of an old home foundation and a couple of aging apple trees left over from a family orchard. On the left (east) side of the trail, the

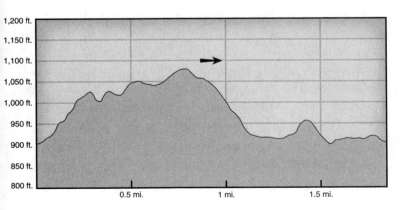

Homesite Trail goes down the hill and, after passing an old house foundation, arrives at the bottom of the Ridge Trail. As the Homesite Trail goes left, the Ridge Trail changes to the Meadows Trail by going straight (south)—follow the Meadows Trail. A few steps ahead, take a look to the left and see if you can identify one of the young chestnut trees planted by park management.

The Meadows Trail continues to drop in elevation, leading to a wide field with dogwood trees and brushy piles of tight vegetation. Deer and coyotes share this field for both feeding and roaming—come early to capture a wall-hanging-worthy photo. At 1.2 miles the trail crosses a 40-foot bridge over a healthy-looking stream. Don't hurry across; stop and watch the water closely to see how many aquatic critters you can spot moving through the riffles and back into a pool. If you want to know more about stream life, there is an interpretive sign detailing just that for your review. The meadow opens up even more to the right as the trail turns back north toward the starting point. A second bridge re-crosses the creek 0.2 mile after the initial crossing.

At the 1.5-mile mark, the Meadows Trail meets the Ridge Trail (straight), and the Homesite Trail comes down to meet the main trails from the left—continue north on the Ridge Trail. The contour of the ridge bottom leads onward to the parking areas. The first one you reach (at 1.6 miles) is accessible from the spur trail joining the Ridge Trail. This area also features the Springhouse Program Area and picnic shelters. At that spur trail junction is another map sign just like the one you saw at the start of this hike. The trail now heads back under tree cover but offers nearly flat walking, not heart-pumping hill climbing. This fine hike ends 0.2 mile ahead.

Nearby Attractions

Historical Canal Winchester is only 3 miles to the northwest of Chestnut Ridge Metro Park. The Ohio and Erie Canal passed through the town and was used for nearly 50 years in the late 1800s. Explore downtown Canal Winchester, as several buildings and homes are on the National Register of Historic Places. Sit on a street-side patio and enjoy lunch or dinner in this quaint village.

Directions

From I-270, take US 33 east 11.3 miles and turn right on Winchester Road. Travel 2.8 miles to the park entrance on the left.

Clear Creek Metro Park

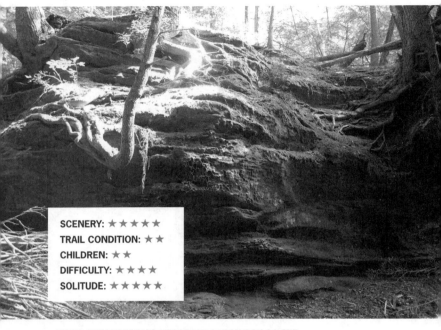

SCENERY: ★ ★ ★ ★ ★
TRAIL CONDITION: ★ ★
CHILDREN: ★ ★
DIFFICULTY: ★ ★ ★
SOLITUDE: ★ ★ ★ ★ ★

ROCK OUTCROPPINGS DECORATE A HEMLOCK RAVINE.

GPS TRAILHEAD COORDINATES: N39° 35.337' W82° 34.667'

DISTANCE & CONFIGURATION: 5-mile loop

HIKING TIME: About 4 hours

HIGHLIGHTS: Hemlock forest, rock outcroppings, ridgetop views

ELEVATION: 783' at trailhead; 1,141' at highest point

ACCESS: Year-round, daily, 6:30 a.m.–sunset

MAPS: At bulletin boards and **tinyurl.com/clearcreekpark**

FACILITIES: Restroom, drinking water, picnic areas

WHEELCHAIR ACCESS: No

COMMENTS: The park is a state nature preserve, so you may not collect any plant, animal, or other substance. Pets are prohibited on these trails, although pet trails are available elsewhere in the park.

CONTACTS: 185 Clear Creek Road, Rockbridge, OH 43149; 614-891-0700; **tinyurl.com/clearcreekpark**

Overview

Walk through a creekside meadow of wildflowers to reach the start of a 4-mile stretch of seclusion and serenity. After climbing a steep switchback to the ridgetop, cruise along a mowed service road. Views of neighboring ridges sporadically open up on both sides of the forested crest trail before you descend into a mature hemlock forest. Maneuver around and over mossy boulders through the thick forest, before bursting out of the woods to follow the Clear Creek once again. This hike includes the Cemetery Ridge, Hemlock, and Creekside Meadows Trails.

Route Details

If the success of a nature preserve is judged by the quality and quantity of its flora and fauna, then Clear Creek Metro Park scores an A-plus. One reason for this high score is that Clear Creek's 5,300 acres are the most studied in the state by professional and amateur naturalists. The extra attention makes it tough for interesting plants and animals to go unnoticed; however, the nature preserve is never crowded. During this 5-mile adventure, I passed only one other pair of hikers—and this was late on a beautiful Saturday morning. Another reason the preserve earns high marks is its rural location and the strict enforcement of regulations. Animals are protected at Clear Creek, and the habitat is not damaged but well managed. And the best part: 20-plus miles of hiking trails provide in-depth exposure to this natural paradise—it's my favorite hike in the book.

The park has four picnic areas; you'll encounter the first, Creekside Meadows Picnic Area, on the drive in from US 33. The Creekside Meadows Trail runs through it, following Clear Creek for 1.7 miles. Take this trail to the east from the picnic area parking lot. Waltzing along the mowed path through a meadow of mixed wildflowers is a nice warm-up for the ridge you are about to climb. Only 0.2 mile from the parking lot, a trail sign will direct you to make a left turn, walk a couple hundred feet, and cross Clear Creek Road to

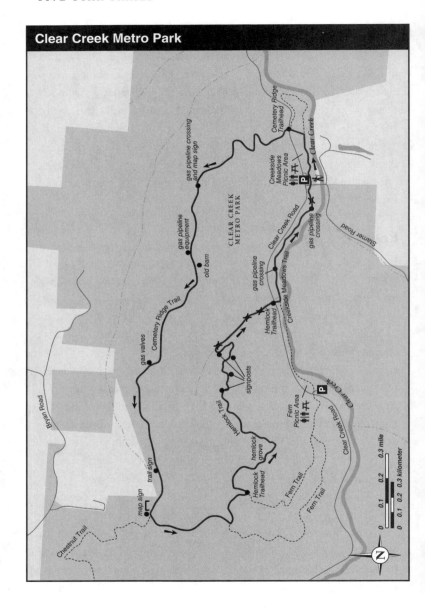

Clear Creek Metro Park

CLEAR CREEK
METRO PARK

Cemetery Ridge Trailhead

Clear Creek

Creekside Meadows Picnic Area

gas pipeline crossing and map sign

Clear Creek Road

gas pipeline crossing

Stamer Road

Creekside Meadows Trail

gas pipeline equipment

old barn

gas pipeline crossing

Cemetery Ridge Trail

Hemlock Trailhead

gas valves

Hemlock Trail

signposts

Fern Picnic Area

Clear Creek

Bryan Road

Clear Creek Road

trail sign

hemlock grove

Hemlock Trailhead

Fern Trail

Fern Trail

map sign

Chestnut Trail

Fern Trail

0   0.1   0.2   0.3 mile
0 0.1 0.2 0.3 kilometer

N

the Cemetery Ridge Trailhead. Cemetery Ridge Trail enters the woods and immediately starts to climb. Four segments of switchbacks gain just over 200 feet in about 0.25 mile. At the top, the forest opens up with larger trees providing large canopies. The packed dirt trail is sprinkled with acorns dropped by white oaks in late summer and early autumn. During years with a good acorn crop, it seems as if you are walking on marbles. The hard little nuts attract deer and turkeys by the dozens, so go slowly around blind corners for a glimpse of wildlife preparing for winter.

The trail breaks out of the full tree cover near the 0.9-mile point, following the ridge, which is also utilized as a maintenance road for a natural gas pipeline. For the next 1.5 miles, the hike follows this ridgetop right-of-way, transitioning from a 20-foot-wide mowed path to crushed limestone tracks. Tall, wide, wooded hollows flank the path. An old barn stands a dozen yards to the south side of the trail at 1.25 miles. The 56-foot, three-bay barn is in surprisingly great condition for being the last remnant of a bustling early 1800s farm. An interpretive sign provides a glimpse into the barn owner's past and explains what life was like in this rugged country a couple of centuries ago.

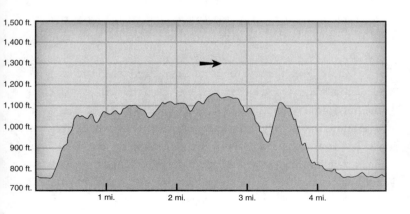

The Cemetery Ridge Trail meets the Chestnut Trail coming into a clearing from the west at 2.5 miles. This mowed area in a meadow features wildflowers, tree saplings, a bench, and a "You Are Here" map sign; trail identification signs point the way. Stay on the Cemetery Ridge Trail as it sneaks off to the south and through a corridor of young hardwoods. Travel down a sloping meadow to meet the Fern Trail, 0.4 mile from the Chestnut Trail junction. Pay close attention to the birds flying about this ridge meadow and do a quick count of the species. The Ohio Audubon Society has recognized the preserve as an Important Birding Area. Take a left on the Fern Trail and wind along a narrow woodland path for 0.3 mile to the upper trailhead of the Hemlock Trail—the paramount section of this hike.

For 1.5 miles, you will pass through—as the name hints— hemlock groves lining rugged ravines. The aromatic trees, along with the moss-decorated, rocky, deep ravines cutting up the ridge, create the sensation you are treading in a mystical place. The Hemlock Trail is not all downhill. After passing through a young grove, the route turns and climbs straight up a steep ridge. Descending the other side of the crest, the trail winds in and out of outcroppings, slump rocks (boulders that have fallen from cliffs above), and below short cliffs. At the bottom, the trail follows a trickling tributary to Clear Creek. You'll reach the park road at 4.4 miles and cross to join the west section of Creekside Meadows Trail. Head east, the same direction the creek flows.

Clear Creek flows with, as its name suggests, clear water over sandstone bedrock and loose rocks. The valley and ravines were cut by melting glacial waters. The creek water is clean and cool most of the year and is one of only three waterways in the state that can sustain stocked trout. About a dozen fishing access points dot Clear Creek Road, but few anglers actually visit the creek. Creekside Meadows Trail passes near the creek's edge, with views up- and downstream. Look closely at barely submerged logs anchored to shore, as trout and other fish will be hiding behind the wood, waiting on food to float by.

Speaking of food, the Creekside Meadows Picnic Area is just ahead, so consider enjoying your own lunch creekside.

Nearby Attractions

About 3 miles north of Clear Creek Metro Park is an additional opportunity to experience nature at its finest. The Wahkeena Nature Preserve (owned and managed by the Ohio Historical Society) has a variety of wild plants and animals on its 150 acres. The preserve is a classroom for naturalists and also for those who simply want to take a walk among wild things. Programs are scheduled throughout the spring, summer, and fall, focusing on subjects such as wildflowers, insects, aquatic life, reptiles, and the habitat that supports it all. The preserve's natural features include a pond, meadows, rugged woodlands, a boardwalk, and a nature center with detailed displays. The preserve is open April–October, Wednesday–Sunday, 8 a.m.– 4:30 p.m.; it's closed November–March.

Directions to Wahkeena Nature Preserve: From US 33, north of Clear Creek Road, turn left onto Sharp Road. Bear right at the T in the road as it becomes Old Logan Road. Drive north 0.7 mile to Pump Station Road and turn left. The preserve entrance is 0.8 mile on the right.

Directions

From Columbus, follow US 33 south for 40 miles to Clear Creek Road. Turn right and drive 1.9 miles to the parking lot on the left.

Conkle's Hollow State Nature Preserve

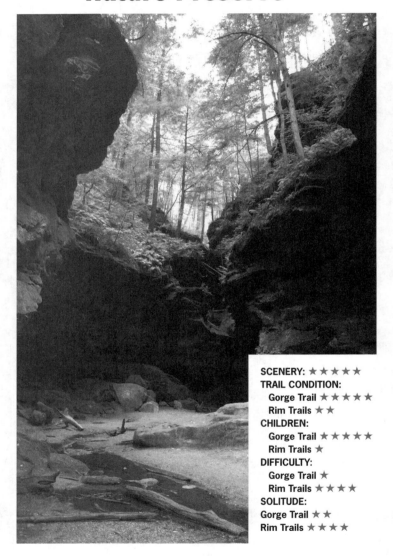

SCENERY: ★ ★ ★ ★ ★
TRAIL CONDITION:
  Gorge Trail ★ ★ ★ ★ ★
  Rim Trails ★ ★
CHILDREN:
  Gorge Trail ★ ★ ★ ★ ★
  Rim Trails ★
DIFFICULTY:
  Gorge Trail ★
  Rim Trails ★ ★ ★ ★
SOLITUDE:
  Gorge Trail ★ ★
  Rim Trails ★ ★ ★ ★

GLACIAL MELTWATERS CARVED THE LANDSCAPE SEEN TODAY, BUT NOW ONLY A TRICKLING CREEK PASSES THROUGH.

GPS TRAILHEAD COORDINATES: N39° 27.211' W82° 34.405'

DISTANCE & CONFIGURATION: 3-mile loop

HIKING TIME: About 2 hours

HIGHLIGHTS: Cliffs, waterfalls

ELEVATION: 731' at trailhead; 1,140' at the highest point

ACCESS: Year-round, daily, sunrise–sunset

MAPS: Posted on bulletin board at trailhead and at **tinyurl.com/chollowmap**

FACILITIES: Restroom

WHEELCHAIR ACCESS: Yes—Gorge Trail is 0.5-mile paved path

COMMENTS: Pets are not allowed in the nature preserve.

CONTACTS: 24858 Big Pine Road, Rockbridge, OH 43149; 614-265-6561; **tinyurl.com/chollow**

Overview

Conkle's Hollow features a fine representation of what the popular Hocking Hills region is all about, and without a lot of company on the trails. Cruise the concrete Gorge Trail up the center of the deep and colorful gorge for an easy walk and awesome view of geological wonders. Return to the gorge entrance, and if you are adventurous and not overly scared of heights, climb the wooden stairway up nearly 200 feet to the edge of the gorge rim. The East and West Rim Trails form a 2-mile loop with several toes-to-the-edge views of the deep hollow below.

Route Details

The Hocking Hills region is home to several geological attractions, but Conkle's Hollow provides a deep look at what the region offers in the ecotourism category. If you are looking to avoid the crowds at Old Man's Cave, then Conkle's Hollow, which is only a few miles away, is a worthy option. Even when Conkle's Hollow is busy, there will be stretches of solitary trail time—even on the paved pathway along the gorge floor.

If the parking area is full, drive down the preserve road to the cul-de-sac and park along the outer edge. The footbridge leading into

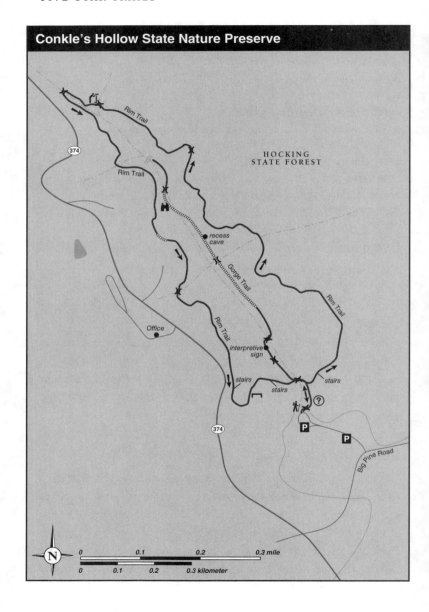

Conkle's Hollow State Nature Preserve

the forest on the north side is the trailhead for both the Gorge and Rim Trails. Wildflowers decorate the woods' edge near the footbridge with species such as the deep-purple spotted knapweed. The heart of the hollow thrives with cool- and moisture-loving vegetation and trees. A boardwalk on the Gorge Trail picks up the guiding duties on the other side of the bridge and steers hikers into the hollow. A set of bulletin boards provides a great deal of information, as do a few interpretive signs, along the paved Gorge Trail.

The temperature drops several degrees early in the walk, as sunshine struggles to reach into the narrow hollow. Carpets of ferns lie along the hollow floor and climb up cliff faces for several yards, beckoning you into this special place. Ohio's state nature preserves are in financial despair because of funding cuts. Signs of tough economic times are evident in the lack of maintenance on things such as mowing and structural repairs. A box for monetary donations is perched along the paved pathway; if you are so inclined, throw in a buck or two to help retain these special places for future generations.

Small recess caves pock the bases of the towering cliffs at a few points on both sides of the hollow, and slump rocks (boulders

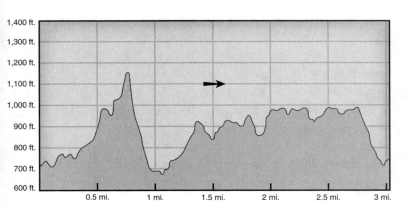

that have fallen from cliffs above) stand along the bases like tanks guarding a fort. As the Gorge Trail nears the head of the hollow and the waterfall, the paving stops and a 3-foot-wide sandy dirt path completes the trek. The trail climbs over rock debris that has fallen from the cliffs over thousands of years. Finally, the hollow's largest waterfall appears between rock ledges. Sound easily bounces off the hollow walls, echoing any noise when someone approaches— certainly this was an advantage for the American Indians who used the hollow as a refuge at times.

Turn around and return to the two flights of stairs near the hollow entrance; one flight leads up each side to the top of the rim. This is where you have to decide whether or not to attempt the East and West Rim Trails. Multiple signs near the stairs and on the way up warn hikers that the Rim Trails are not for the weak or those scared of heights. I'm no fan of heights, but I made the climb to the East Rim and soon was huffing and puffing—not all because of the steep climb. The thought of standing on the edge of a 200-foot cliff edge was sending danger alert signals throughout my mind. But I do love adventure, so I pushed on to the first cliff edge intersection in this rugged 2-mile extension of the Conkle's Hollow tour.

If the stair climb is too much, turn around and go right back down. If you're still energized, however, climb the rooty and rocky trail to the top of the first cliff edge at 1.4 miles (counting the 1 mile completed in the gorge). A few steel stakes with rope serve as a handrail as the trail reaches the rim, but at the top and for the next 0.5 mile there are no safety riggings. It's just you and the cliff edges— watch your step. The East Rim Trail provides better views than the West Rim Trail, but it's also more dangerous. The trail follows the rim very closely, and a couple of open fractures in the cliff top near the edge could injure a hiker's foot and even cause a fatal fall in a second. I can't say it enough: Don't be so obsessed with the views of the distant ridges or the gorge below that you disregard the placement of your next step.

A wooden observation deck greets hikers at the top of the major waterfall seen earlier at the head of the hollow. A fence with wooden rails leads to the creek crossing a dozen yards upstream and over to the West Rim Trail. This path also follows the cliff edge but without as many overlooks, although you can sense that the woodland you are walking in drops off sharply to your left. At 2.25 miles you will cross a small stream simply by walking on the bedrock of the creek. During wet periods, this crossing can become a sliding board with a deadly landing, as the cliff edge is only a couple of yards from the trail at that point. Just 0.5 mile down the trail a similar creek crossing also requires caution. The long set of stairs at the beginning was a warm-up for the descent at the south end of the West Rim Trail. A set of wood-and-stone steps delivers you back to the paved Gorge Trail near the mouth of the hollow.

Nearby Attractions

About 4 miles north of Conkle's Hollow on OH 374 is another rock formation accessible by a short but demanding hiking trail. Rock House is a true natural cave, complete with openings like windows overlooking a wooded valley. The Rock House doesn't feel confining, as the cave is not deep in the rock hillside but instead is spread out over 200 feet across a cliff face. The cave ceiling is about 20 feet high, and space between walls is nearly 30 feet, creating the house-like formation. The 0.5-mile hiking trail has a picnic shelter and a latrine.

Directions

From I-270, follow US 33 south 36 miles to OH 180. Drive south on OH 180 for 3.5 miles to OH 678. Continue south on OH 678 for 4 miles to OH 374. Follow OH 374 south 3.4 miles to Big Pine Road on the left. Drive past the church to the park entrance on the left.

Hocking Hills
State Park: Old Man's Cave

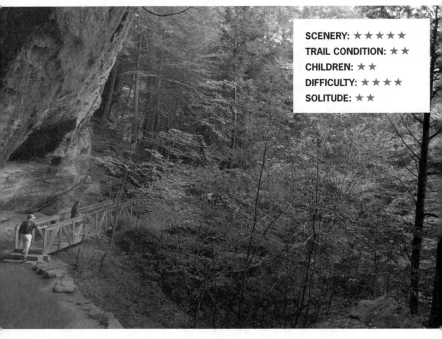

SCENERY: ★ ★ ★ ★ ★
TRAIL CONDITION: ★ ★
CHILDREN: ★ ★
DIFFICULTY: ★ ★ ★ ★
SOLITUDE: ★ ★

CLIFF WALLS CONTAIN MOST OF THE HIKE AT OLD MAN'S CAVE.

GPS TRAILHEAD COORDINATES: N39° 26.170' W82° 32.339'

DISTANCE & CONFIGURATION: 5.7-mile loop

HIKING TIME: About 4 hours

HIGHLIGHTS: Caves, cliffs, waterfalls

ELEVATION: 784' at trailhead; 1,082' at highest point

ACCESS: Year-round, daily, sunrise–sunset

MAPS: At visitor center, bulletin boards, and **tinyurl.com/hhparkmap**

FACILITIES: Restrooms, water, visitor center, picnic areas

WHEELCHAIR ACCESS: No; yes at nearby Ash Cave

COMMENTS: Pets must be leashed. Young children should be closely supervised.

CONTACTS: 19852 OH 664 S., Logan, OH 43138; 740-385-6842; **tinyurl.com/hhpark**

Overview

Walk through a gorge with some of Ohio's most-visited geological wonders at Hocking Hills State Park. Follow Grandma Gatewood's Trail past Old Man's Cave and several impressive rock formations created by water and time. This popular trail crosses a few bridges and pauses at a few waterfalls. As it distances itself from the visitor center, the crowds vanish. Climb over rocks and up, down, and through fallen cliff boulders on the way to Cedar Creek Falls—the turnaround point. Return to the heavily visited cave via the Gorge Overlook Trail while passing by a remote trout lake.

Route Details

About 350 million years ago, Ohio was covered by an ancient sea. Sandstone was created by compressing and settling sand at the bottom of the old sea. Some of that rock became a harder stone within the layers of compressed sandstone. Glacial waters and other eroding forces erased the softer layers from the harder layers, creating caverns of various shapes and sizes. Recess caves are the most common, with the harder stone on top creating a cave roof and an empty space where the now-eroded softer stone once was. Those spaces, including Old Man's Cave, have become the focus of stories and legends passed from generation to generation. Now they attract thousands of annual visitors as well. Hiking through these gorges and caves never gets old—and neither does the lore.

This detailed hike starts at the visitor center on the cliff tops above Old Man's Cave. Resist the urge to grab an ice cream cone before you begin. Take the sidewalk north past the picnic shelter and look for the cliff warning sign on the right. Cross a bridge over Old Man's Creek and admire the plunge pool created 40 feet below the upper falls. Grandma Gatewood's Trail turns right and passes only a few feet from the edge of the drop. There will be many more close encounters with cliff edges—if children are along for this hike, exercise extreme caution and watch them closely. Take the flight of

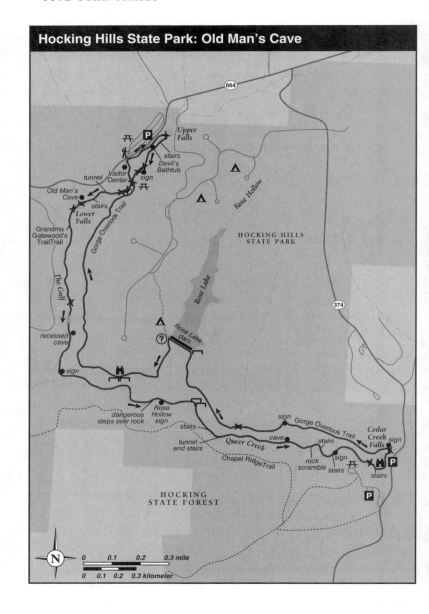

Hocking Hills State Park: Old Man's Cave

664

Upper Falls

stairs
Devil's Bathtub

tunnel

Visitor Center

sign

Old Man's Cave

stairs

Lower Falls

Grandma Gatewood's Trail Trail

Gorge Overlook Trail

Rose Hollow

HOCKING HILLS STATE PARK

The Gulf

Rose Lake

374

recessed cave

sign

Rose Lake dam

?

dangerous steps over rock

Rose Hollow sign

stairs

tunnel and stairs

Chapel Ridge Trail

Queer Creek

sign

cave

Gorge Overlook Trail

stairs

Cedar Creek Falls

sign

rock scramble

sign

stairs

stairs

P

HOCKING STATE FOREST

P

N

0   0.1   0.2   0.3 mile
0   0.1   0.2   0.3 kilometer

stairs to the right and descend to the gorge floor near the plunge pool. For the next 0.5 mile you will follow the gorge south, observing some of the most interesting rock formations in the world. Nine footbridges jump the creek back and forth along this stretch, passing by sights such as Devil's Bathtub, Sphinx Head, and, of course, Old Man's Cave.

Grandma Gatewood's Trail is also a section of the Buckeye Trail, or BT to avid Ohio hikers. It's a 1,444-mile hiking route that loops around Ohio, nearly touching all four corners. The BT is identified with blue blazes, markings approximately 2 inches wide and 6 inches long painted on trees, to guide hikers. On the trip from Old Man's Cave to Cedar Creek Falls, 6-inch-square posts with a band of blue paint around the top also identify the path as the Buckeye Trail. The route isn't crowded like it is in the main gorge, but it's easily noticeable.

Slump rocks (boulders that have fallen from cliffs above) dot the gorge floor; some even have living trees rooted to them. Mosses cover many of the stones lying around the cool environment created by the gorge. At 1.3 miles, the trail provides a 60-foot boardwalk to level the hiking surface. The trail section from here to Cedar Creek Falls is the most rugged of the route, but it's fun to negotiate. Glance

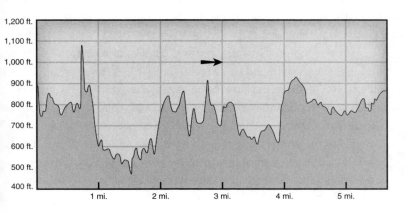

back and forth from one gorge wall to the other to see additional recess caves, narrow waterfalls, and interesting rock piles. Just past the boardwalk is a stand of large hemlock trees, and the trail runs through it—breathe deep and fill those senses. Near the 2-mile point, trail blazes lead up and around a large rock outcropping bordering the creek, 15 feet below. Not many hikers follow the blazes, which return to the creekside trail via steep stone steps on the other side of the outcropping. Instead, a popular shortcut demands hikers to hold tree roots, which are growing down from the outcropping, and side step along a ledge in the rock above the creek bank for about 20 feet to reach the level trail and continue to Cedar Creek Falls.

Several additional run-ins with boulders await, but it's not a tough course for even the average walker—simply watch your footing. The trail gets so close to the cliff base at a few points that you will actually be walking with the cliff overhead. A mason-laid stone wall rises along the creek bank as you near the 3-mile point, which means Cedar Creek Falls is just around the corner. Cross a footbridge over the waterfall's spill-off to reach the lower observation area, which is a great location to enjoy a light lunch. There are two ways up to the top of the falls—the one you want is the series of wooden stairs and deck overlooks closest to the waterfall. The other way up is a long series of steps (the first you come to as you enter the Cedar Creek Falls area) to a paved parking area.

At the top of the stairs, a gravel path leads to a suspension bridge above the falls and by a second Cedar Creek Falls parking lot along OH 374. Cross the suspension bridge and turn left. The trail is a wide road through the woods. Posts with red blazes confirm you're on the Gorge Overlook Trail. At 3.9 miles, the trail climbs 300 feet in 0.3 mile to the pretty, trout-stocked Rose Lake and then crosses the dam. The trail section from the suspension bridge to Rose Lake is less traveled and less dramatic than the creekside trail; enjoy this quiet stretch. From the north side of the dam, the trail turns to the left and downhill; the small path going uphill leads to the campground. At 4.5 miles an overlook, complete with a stone railing and benches, offers a peek into the forested gorge. This rim walk leads to a bridge at the 5.5-mile point that crosses Old Man's Creek and arrives at the visitor center. Now have that ice cream.

Nearby Attractions

Ohio's largest cave, Ash Cave, is 2 miles south of Cedar Creek Falls. The massive cavern measures 700 feet wide, 100 feet deep, and 100 feet tall. A paved, wheelchair-accessible, 0.25-mile pathway leads from the parking area to the cave's plunge pool. A wheelchair-accessible restroom and a picnic area are available at the parking area as well. A 0.5-mile rim trail leaves the paved pathway for a cliff-edge tour of the cave and demands safe hiking practices. The paved pathway leads visitors through a narrow gorge that was cut by the creek water flowing over what is now the cliff roof. Take a camera, take your time, and imagine what the cave looked like a few hundred years ago when American Indians used the natural shelter. From Old Man's Cave parking area, drive north on OH 664 to OH 374. Follow OH 374 south 3.5 miles to OH 56 and turn right. The parking area is on the left, and the cave pathway is on the right.

Directions

From Columbus, follow US 33 south 39 miles to OH 664. Travel south on OH 664 for 10 miles to Old Man's Cave parking lot and trailhead.

Rockbridge State Nature Preserve

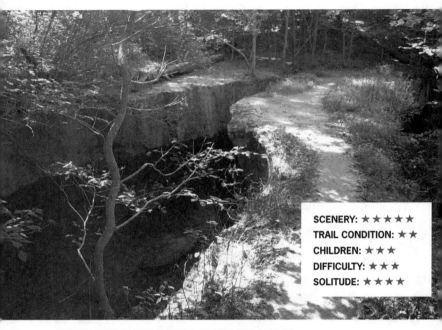

SCENERY: ★ ★ ★ ★ ★
TRAIL CONDITION: ★ ★
CHILDREN: ★ ★ ★
DIFFICULTY: ★ ★ ★
SOLITUDE: ★ ★ ★ ★

TIPTOE ACROSS THIS NATURAL BRIDGE FOR A THRILL.

GPS TRAILHEAD COORDINATES: N39° 33.978' W82° 29.959'

DISTANCE & CONFIGURATION: 2.4-mile balloon

HIKING TIME: About 2 hours

HIGHLIGHTS: Natural bridge, ravines

ELEVATION: 852' at trailhead; 939' at highest point

ACCESS: Year-round, daily, sunrise–sunset

MAPS: At bulletin board at trailhead parking lot

FACILITIES: None

WHEELCHAIR ACCESS: No

COMMENTS: Hikers must remain on trails in Ohio nature preserves. Rockbridge can be crossed on foot, but only with extreme caution.

CONTACTS: 614-265-6561; **tinyurl.com/rockbridgesnp**

Overview

Getting a good look at Ohio's largest natural bridge requires a 1-mile trek along a mowed corridor flanked by brushy field edges. Escape the farm fields and climb up a root- and rock-strewn dirt trail through mixed hardwood forest. Drop over the top of the hill and enter a wooded valley to find the preserve's main feature stretching across a creek ravine nearly out of sight from the trail. Leave the bridge and wind your way up to a neighboring hilltop, with the option to hike the Rock Shelter Trail (an extra 0.75 mile) from the peak. Either way, re-cross the first forest valley to the entry corridor and retrace your steps back to the trailhead.

Route Details

From the trailhead, which sits at the edge of a pasture, there is no sign that you're near an amazing geological feature. Even locating the trailhead and parking lot is a bit tricky (see Directions on page 179). Once you convince yourself that the small, paved parking lot with only a dozen spaces is the place, approach the sheltered bulletin board next to the last parking space to begin the hike. A mowed, 12-foot-wide corridor running between a pasture on the left and a tree row bordering a hayfield on the right is the pathway to the heart of the nature preserve. Two boardwalks skim over a couple of wet areas between the fields before you climb the hill to the preserve's woodland. Early-morning hikers may get a glimpse of deer grazing in the hayfield.

The trail leaves the fields and enters the woods at 0.4 mile. Exposed tree roots run across the trail, providing traction on the steep dirt path. Rain can really create a problem on the scramble to the top, so if there is a reason to don the raingear, include a hiking pole or two. A bench sits between the trail and pasture fence at the top of the knoll for a quick break. At 0.5 mile the trail splits. This is the beginning of the Natural Bridge Trail—marked with an orange arrow badge at signposts along the trail. A blue arrow badge identifies the

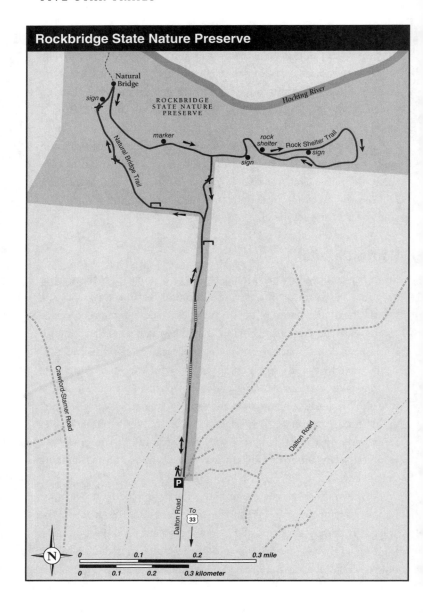

Rockbridge State Nature Preserve

Natural Bridge

sign

ROCKBRIDGE STATE NATURE PRESERVE

Hocking River

marker

rock shelter

Rock Shelter Trail

sign

Natural Bridge Trail

sign

Crawford-Starner Road

Dalton Road

Dalton Road

P

To 33

N

0   0.1   0.2   0.3 mile

0   0.1   0.2   0.3 kilometer

Rock Shelter Trail, which is accessed from the Natural Bridge Trail. Take the narrow trail to the left that runs parallel with the pasture fence up the hill.

The young woods and underbrush lean in close to the trail for the next 0.25 mile. A stony-bottomed creek comes next as the hillside begins to level out. At 0.8 mile the trail arrives at an intersection. The path leading off to the right is the continuation of the Natural Bridge Trail. The route to the left is the way to the natural bridge, which is just around the bend to the left. Signposts at that point will confirm the directions. Keep a close eye on the trail's edge as you approach the bridge, as a few crevices in the bedrock reach out near the path. There are no safety rails or ropes to prevent a fall if you get too close to the edge.

The natural bridge measures 100 feet long by 10 feet wide and arches 50 feet over the creek below—it's an impressive piece of Ohio's geology. The bridge is accessible for those who want to cross to the other side. *Note:* A thin covering of soil coats the center of the bridge, and it can quickly turn to mud on wet days. But for the best view, take the curving path down around and underneath the bridge

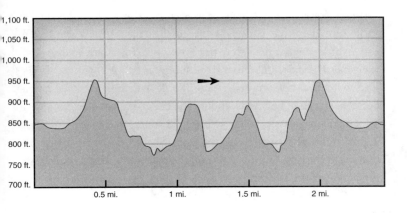

to the floor of what was a total recess cave. The bridge, created by the fall of the center section of the recess cave, is actually the remaining front edge of the cave roof. The creek the trail was following before arriving at the bridge now flows over the cave's "skylight" and falls between the cave and the bridge.

It's difficult to simply glimpse the bridge and immediately continue the hike. Plan at least 20 minutes or more to explore and take in the site. Another spur trail breaks off of the under-bridge access trail and leads to the Hocking River, a few hundred feet downstream. Paddlers often take a break from the river fun to hike up and admire the natural bridge. While hanging out here you may hear laughing, a few screams, and an odd zinging sound on the neighboring ridge, rising from the opposite side of the bridge. That's all coming from ziplines and the high-flying passengers at the Hocking Hills Canopy Tours, which is particularly busy on weekends during the summer months.

Return to the intersection and follow the access trail up the hill and across the ridge to meet the optional Rock Shelter Trail. It soon becomes apparent by the thin path that this trail is often bypassed by visitors to the natural bridge. The name, Rock Shelter, likely brings thoughts of a recess cave protecting a group of American Indians or settlers. Not so much. It's a small recess cave, and a group of slump rocks (boulders that have fallen from cliffs above) now sits in the center of a deep ravine below the little cave. The Rock Shelter Trail traverses a hillside, still under tree canopy, as is this entire route. The trail switchbacks downward, stopping a dozen yards from the ravine bottom, and then begins ascending the hill at a lower elevation, with 4-inch square posts guiding you. At 1.3 miles, and before reaching a small footbridge, you'll see the Rock Shelter down in the ravine bottom to the left. You must stay on the path, and no spur trail exists for exploring the shelter.

Cross the footbridge and amble up through a hardwood forest to a trail sign. Follow the 0.25-mile loop around the woods and begin the return trek down past the shelter and back up the path to rejoin the Natural Bridge Trail. Cross the wooded valley you traveled through on the way to the natural bridge, and in 0.1 mile you'll arrive at the trail you came in on. Retrace your route up the little rise along the forest edge and down the mowed corridor to the parking area.

Nearby Attractions

The remote Cantwell Cliffs stand about 4 miles to the southwest of Rockbridge State Nature Preserve on OH 374. A 1-mile hiking trail explores the tops and the bottoms of the cliffs and the surrounding forest. Several narrow trail passages allow visitors to get close to the sandstone walls and huge chunks of rock. Rim trails circle the cliff tops with views that are especially attractive during the colorful leaf-changing season.

Directions

From I-270 travel US 33 south 35 miles to Dalton Road. Turn left and follow Dalton Road 0.7 mile to the parking lot and trailhead on the left.

27

Shallenberger State Nature Preserve

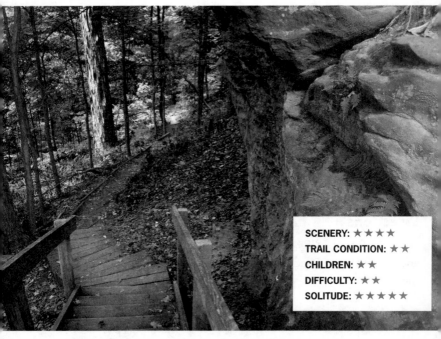

SCENERY: ★ ★ ★ ★
TRAIL CONDITION: ★ ★
CHILDREN: ★ ★
DIFFICULTY: ★ ★
SOLITUDE: ★ ★ ★ ★ ★

WOOD STAIRS ASSIST HIKERS TO THE TOP OF THE ROCKY RIDGE.

GPS TRAILHEAD COORDINATES: N39º 41.492' W82º 39.421'

DISTANCE & CONFIGURATION: 1.6-mile loop

HIKING TIME: About 1 hour

HIGHLIGHTS: Preserved woodland, distant views, rock outcroppings

ELEVATION: 1,007' at trailhead; 1,139' at highest point

ACCESS: Open a half hour before sunrise to a half hour after sunset

MAPS: tinyurl.com/shallenbergersnp

FACILITIES: None

WHEELCHAIR ACCESS: No

COMMENTS: No pets or bikes allowed. Allen Knob Trail passes near a cliff edge—stay on the trail.

CONTACTS: 614-265-6561; tinyurl.com/shallenbergersnp

Overview

Enter at the base of the tallest of the two forest-covered, rocky knobs and remain under tree canopy for the entire hike. Circle the knob base and then climb a steep spur trail for a view from the top. Return to the main trail and cross a shallow ravine to reach the second smaller knob. A pleasant forest walk among old and young trees swings out and along the northern border of the nature preserve. Before rejoining the main trail near the trailhead, a glance up at the big rocky knob reveals its massive sandstone heart.

Route Details

Father Time and Mother Nature sculpted the two rising features of this state nature preserve. The process started with an ancient sea 300 million years ago, and then just 10,000 years ago a glacier put the finishing touches on what are known as Allen and Ruble Knobs. These two sandstone bumps standing above glaciated flat agricultural fields are covered with a deciduous forest, hiding the natural artwork. But once you enter the forest, it soon becomes evident that the 88-acre nature preserve is bustling with life—some rare, so be alert. Don't let the tranquility of the place dampen your senses.

Although the parking lot accommodates only 16 vehicles, parking is not a problem because this gem of a preserve gets little visitation. From the paved lot in the southwest corner of the property, walk east across a mowed lawn to the tree line to find the trailhead and bulletin board sitting just inside the woods. Also at this point, a plaque set in stone honors the donor and 1973 dedication of the property. Take a few minutes to review the seasonal postings displayed on the bulletin board to ensure you don't miss something naturally special while meandering along the quiet trail.

About 100 feet past the bulletin board, a trail joins from the left. This hike plan will bring you back here on this trail at hike's end. A car-sized stone sits at an angle a few steps up that left-hand trail and provides a close-up look at thousands of years of erosion from

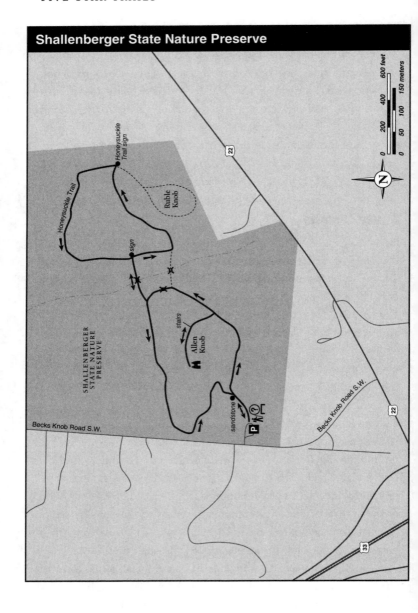

Shallenberger State Nature Preserve

the weather. Follow the trail straight ahead and watch for a buck to rise from its bed in the bottomland to the right of the trail. With bountiful agricultural fields sprawled out around the preserve, white-tailed deer consider the tranquil area a safe zone. Shallenberger State Nature Preserve shows how a section of land can be successfully maintained with regulations and wise management practices. Once you're immersed in the nature preserve's environment, the only reminder of the bustling world outside is the sound of vehicles traveling on US 33.

During my hike here, I witnessed rare burying beetles working on and in the small carcass of a shrew. The black-and-orange, 1-inch-long beetles were doing their dirty work on the trail's edge—watch your step along the narrow dirt path. At 0.2 mile a spur leading to the top of Allen Knob veers off to the left. The steep incline finishes near the top with a set of wooden steps. Before reaching the steps, be cautious of the steel bars protruding a few inches from the ground that once held a now-missing step. The steps wind around a sandstone cliff face, with fluffs of ferns rooted in the cliff's fractures. During late summer, slow-moving giant millipedes can be seen scaling the rocks and trails here.

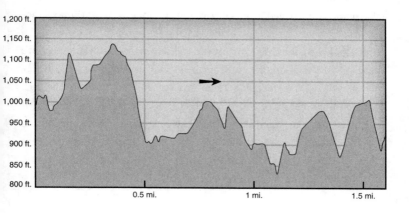

On the peak of Allen Knob, a trail circles the top without any safety rails or cables. If a child is along for this hike, hold his or her hand to avoid accidental falls from the stone cliff edges. The knob top is forested with various tree species, including the rocky-ridge-loving chestnut oak, identified by deeply grooved bark. Also growing on the Virginia Highlands–type rocky soil is a healthy collection of mountain laurels. You'll get the best long-distance views of Lancaster and the Hocking Hills from this tallest knob when the trees are without leaves. Enjoy the ever-present breeze flowing over the knobs.

Back on the main trail and traveling northeast downhill to the 0.6-mile point, a path leads off to the right—take that across a small creek via a wooden footbridge. Then ascend a small rise to the western base of Ruble Knob and the trail that circles the northern side of the knob. Turn right on the trail, and at 0.9 mile find a brown wooden trail sign pointing to the left (north) labeled HONEYSUCKLE TRAIL. Following this route simply continues the loop back to where you turned right after crossing the last bridge. Standing at the Honeysuckle Trail sign, a fading path to the south leads up to the top of Ruble Knob—take that if you want, but don't expect cliff edges or impressive views.

Follow the Honeysuckle Trail through a healthy forest back to the point you arrived at after crossing the long bridge; then retrace your steps back across the bridge to the trail you came in on. Turn right, and the trail leads you around to the north side of Allen Knob's base and runs into the entry trail on the west side of the knob. While walking the west side, take time to pause and admire the rock outcroppings near the top of Allen Knob, and the huge chunks of rock that have tumbled down over the centuries. Mosses and ferns now cover and dress up the stones, enhancing the impressive nature show. The trail winds around the car-sized stone seen at the beginning of the hike. The parking lot is to the right.

Nearby Attractions

The Hocking River has been an asset to thousands of families for centuries in the Lancaster region. During the 1800s, the river's flow was harnessed to spin the wheels of several mills. One has been restored and offers an accurate look at a historic piece of equipment in action. The Rock Mill and Covered Bridge sit on the Hocking River about 6 miles to the northwest of Shallenberger State Nature Preserve. Follow Beck's Knob Road north 2.5 miles to West Fair Avenue. Turn left and soon West Fair Avenue changes to Wilson Road. Travel 2.9 miles and turn right on Mt. Zion Road. Drive 0.9 mile north to Lithopolis Road and turn left. The mill and covered bridge are just ahead on the left. Admire the river there as it plunges nearly 100 feet to a gorge floor.

Directions

From Columbus, follow US 33 south 29 miles to the US 22 exit. Turn left on US 22 and travel east 200 yards to Becks Knob Road. Turn left and drive 0.2 mile to the parking lot on the right.

28

Slate Run Metro Park

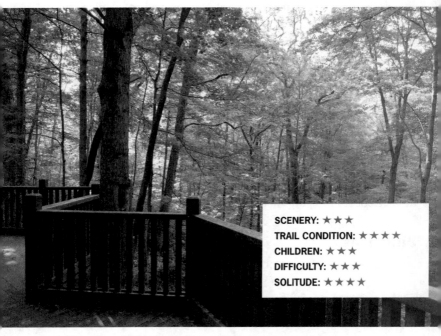

SCENERY: ★ ★ ★
TRAIL CONDITION: ★ ★ ★ ★
CHILDREN: ★ ★ ★
DIFFICULTY: ★ ★ ★
SOLITUDE: ★ ★ ★ ★

OVERLOOK A FORESTED RAVINE FROM THIS OBSERVATION DECK.

GPS TRAILHEAD COORDINATES: N39° 45.528' W82° 50.313'

DISTANCE & CONFIGURATION: 2.2-mile balloon

HIKING TIME: About 2 hours

HIGHLIGHTS: Forested ravine, creek access

ELEVATION: 935' at trailhead; 634' at lowest point

ACCESS: Daily, 6:30 a.m.–sunset

MAPS: At bulletin boards in parking areas, **tinyurl.com/slaterun**

FACILITIES: Restrooms, drinking fountains, playgrounds, picnic areas

WHEELCHAIR ACCESS: Not on detailed trails, but on Lake Trail

COMMENTS: Explore the creek and a wooded hillside in the 7-acre Natural Play Area, accessed from the Shady Grove Picnic Area. Follow Five Oaks Trail past the ravine overlook deck and down to the bottom of the hill. Natural Play Area signs are posted.

CONTACTS: 1375 OH 674 N., Canal Winchester, OH 43110; 614-891-0700; **tinyurl.com/slaterun**

Overview

Start at a quiet picnic area and disappear into the forest, pausing at an observation deck overlooking a steep ravine and a winding creek. Descend to cross the creek and explore the aquatic oasis before climbing to the top on the opposing side. Walk among mixed hardwoods of various ages, then hike back down to the creek for another crossing, and another, and another, before ascending the ridge and returning to the observation deck and finally the picnic area. This hike follows the Five Oaks and Sugar Maple Trails.

Route Details

The geography of central Ohio offers a few surprises for first-time visitors, as the farmlands southeast of Columbus are interrupted by occasional patches of forest and waterways. Slate Run Metro Park is one such patch—quite a patch, actually, at more than 1,700 acres, half wooded. The park's lands were first thought to be sitting on slate, but it was soon discovered the underlying rock was shale, not slate. The area also hides a deep ravine under a canopy of hardwood trees, and that will be our targeted hiking area. The park also offers additional landscapes to investigate, such as meadows, wetlands, and grasslands. Plan to spend half a day and consider one of the two picnic areas to do lunch—or supper if you get a late start.

To access the Shady Grove Picnic Area, take the second left after entering the park's main entrance on OH 674. If possible, park at the western edge of the picnic area. The Five Oaks Trail trailhead is next to the restrooms. The 8-foot-wide crushed limestone path is well maintained, even on steeper stretches. Just as you get started, the picturesque ravine cuts down several yards to the right of the trail. The ravine is forested, but not enough to restrict a decent peek. It widens, and just in time an observation deck provides a wide view of the ravine and the creek that cut it into the landscape. The deck is only 0.2 mile from the trailhead.

Slate Run Metro Park

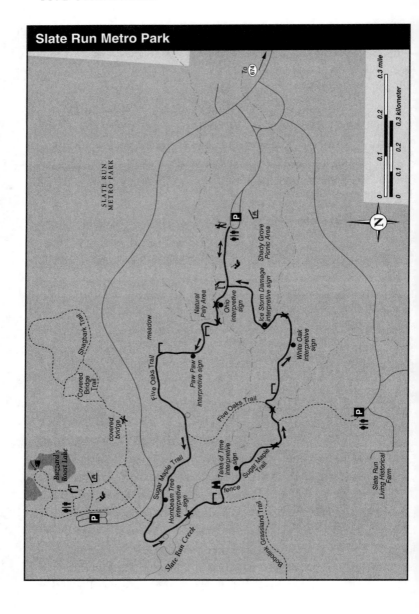

Take the trail to the right and down a steep grade with a split rail fence separating you from the ravine edge. Pause and look back at the shale cliff below the observation deck to see how the creek has carved through the landscape. As you cross the creek on a wooden footbridge, a plunge pool with a small waterfall offers soothing music to the ears. Follow the creek downstream to the designated Natural Play Area, where kids can wade in the shallow water and flip over rocks in search of crawdads and other aquatic life. If you can pull your young hiker (or yourself) from the play area, make your way back to the trail, which begins to rise quickly up the north side of the ravine. At 0.4 mile a bench provides a welcome sight after the steep climb out of the creek bed. A few wide-trunked beech trees stand near the trail and easily lure the mind into wondering what it was like here a couple hundred years ago.

The trail breaks free of the forest for a few steps with a view of a designated conservation area. But back into the woods you go and down to the creek again, walking through a brushy stand of saplings. At 0.75 mile the Five Oaks Trail turns to the left and the Sugar Maple Trail goes straight. Continuing west, take the Sugar Maple option.

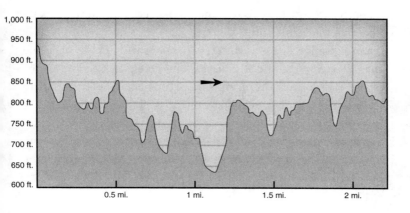

Several interpretive signs note different tree species, which should strengthen your forestry knowledge. A spur off to the right at the 1-mile point leads to the Buzzard's Roost Lake picnic area.

The Sugar Maple Trail turns back to the east and crosses the creek again on a bridge. Then up the hill you go. A demanding jaunt to the top of the ravine gets the blood flowing, but no worries, as a bench waits at the top. At 1.25 miles the Bobolink Grassland Trail turns off to the right. The Bobolink connects to the Kokomo Wetland Trail to create a nice side trip. Be sure you have an extra two hours if you want to add that to your itinerary. The Sugar Maple Trail swings out along the ridge edge to a fenced observation point overlooking the widening ravine. The hike continues around the side of the ridge with a couple of small bridges crossing creek tributaries. Listen for woodpeckers at this point, as the sound of beaks pounding trees easily carries.

At 1.5 miles a spur takes off to the right and leads 500 feet to the Slate Run Living Historical Farm. The working exhibit includes displays of farm life from the 1880s (call 614-833-1880 for seasonal hours). Just 0.1 mile from the farm spur trail, the Sugar Maple Trail meets the Five Oaks Trail—turn right on the Five Oaks Trail and go southeast. After making the turn and hiking to the top of the ridge, a bench and a massive four-trunked oak tree stand near the path. This trail was named after this tree (now missing the fifth trunk). An interpretive sign tells the story. Head on around the ridge and then downhill to a bridge, a pleasant place to pause and watch the pretty stream falling from small pool to small pool on its way to the main creek. The trail slips along a shallow gully bottom and then quickly does a switchback up to the next ridgetop. At 2.1 miles you're back to the observation deck. Take a right and your thorough hike of this beautiful ravine is about finished, but I bet you'll be back for another round.

Nearby Attractions

Chestnut Ridge Metro Park (preserving what is considered the first ridge in the foothills of the Appalachian Mountains) is 2 miles to the northeast. Take a hiking trail to an observation deck perched high on the park's signature ridge, which offers a view of the Columbus skyline.

Directions

From I-270, take US 33 east 5.5 miles to OH 674. Turn right onto OH 674/Gender Road and travel south 2.5 miles to Lithopolis Road. Turn left and go 0.7 mile to OH 674. Turn right and drive 4 miles to the entrance on the right.

Stage's Pond
State Nature Preserve

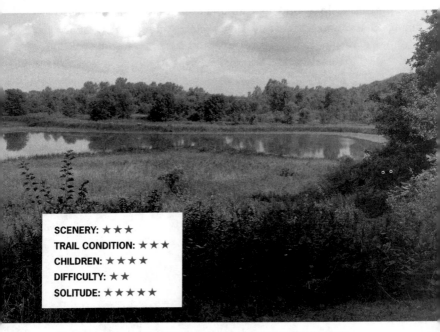

SCENERY: ★ ★ ★
TRAIL CONDITION: ★ ★ ★
CHILDREN: ★ ★ ★ ★
DIFFICULTY: ★ ★
SOLITUDE: ★ ★ ★ ★ ★

A KETTLE LAKE TAKES CENTER STAGE AT THIS NATURE PRESERVE.

GPS TRAILHEAD COORDINATES: N39° 40.211' W82° 56.054'

DISTANCE & CONFIGURATION: 2.4-mile loop

HIKING TIME: About 1.5 hours

HIGHLIGHTS: Kettle (glacial) lake, wildlife observation

ELEVATION: 720' at trailhead, with no significant rise

ACCESS: Year-round, daily, sunrise–sunset

MAPS: At bulletin board at trailhead and **stagespondnaturepreserve.info**

FACILITIES: None

WHEELCHAIR ACCESS: No

COMMENTS: No pets permitted (except assistance animals) on trails. No collection of any plant, animal, or other substance permitted. Visitors are required to stay on trails.

CONTACTS: 4792 Hagerty Road, Ashville, OH 43103; 614-265-6561; **ohiodnr.com/dnap**

Overview

The trails at this out-of-the-way state nature preserve are also less traveled, creating a true wildlife sanctuary. Near the parking lot, you can access a level spur trail to a waterfowl blind. A walk around the perimeter of an old meadow leads to a second blind watching over a kettle lake. A young, brushy forest is popular among birders, and the trail that infiltrates it has a few benches trailside for bird-watching. The preserve is surrounded by agricultural fields, which also attract wildlife. Migrating waterfowl flying over central Ohio often stop here to refuel.

Route Details

The 174-acre Stage's Pond State Nature Preserve sits in the middle of farm country. It's one of Ohio's least-visited nature preserves, simply because it is a few miles off the beaten path. But if you are a wildlife enthusiast, Stage's Pond is a happening place, especially during waterfowl migrations. A kettle lake surrounded by a blend of meadows and woodlands provides plenty of edges for wildlife to jump from food source to cover in short order. What the preserve lacks in natural attractions, it makes up for with an abundance of animal, insect, bird, and wildflower species.

There are two parking areas, and you can access both from the entrance on Hagerty Road on the south side of the preserve. The larger of the two areas is up the paved lane near the preserve office—no facilities for the public. The smaller area is near the preserve entrance. Park at the small lot and you can avoid spooking animals, upping your chance for some wildlife observation. A short walk from the parking area up the lane leads to a footbridge over a drainage ditch and onward to the bulletin board with maps. From there, take the spur trail through a pine grove to reach a substantial observation blind near the edge of a pond. The wooden observation blind is equipped with waterfowl identification posters, just in case you left your bird guidebook behind. With few human visitors to the

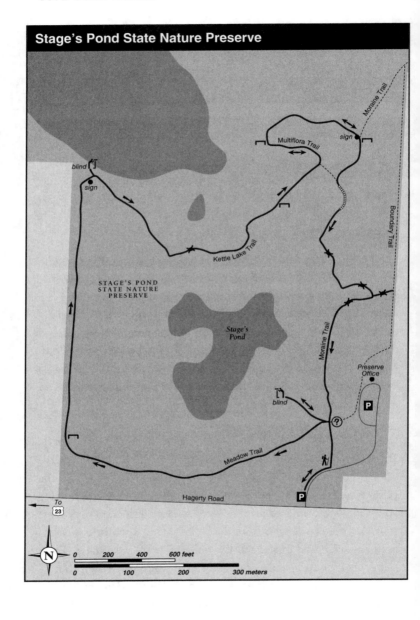

Stage's Pond State Nature Preserve

blind, you'll be surprised at the photo ops the ducks, geese, herons, and shorebirds offer throughout the day.

Return to the bulletin board and follow the Meadow Trail to the south and west. The meadow is sprinkled with various young trees, including some cedars, attempting to reclaim the open land back to forest. Prior to the property becoming a nature preserve, the land was farmed. While there are no signs of farming now, a dedicated and successful land management plan are in order just the same. A wide, mowed pathway follows the south and west boundaries, with a farm field and tree row standing between the preserve and the neighboring property. And because of the preserve's two lakes and marshlands, summer brings a population of dragonflies and damselflies, which regularly buzz along the trail. A bench waits at 0.6 mile—a perfect location to pause for a few moments and see how many butterfly species you can identify.

The Meadow Trail ends just short of the south shore of the 30-acre kettle lake. A kettle lake is a depression in the Earth's surface that was created when a huge chunk of melting glacier fell to the ground. A short spur path turns left off the Kettle Lake Trail,

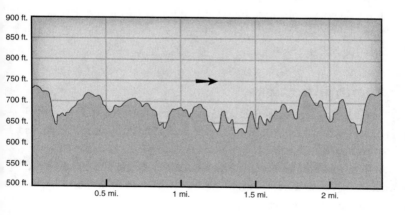

which began at the point the Meadow Trail ended, and leads to a small wood-framed observation blind. These blinds are great spots for getting kids involved in birding and simply being outside more. The preserve would be a pleasant place to enjoy a picnic, but as with all of Ohio's state nature preserves, picnicking is permitted only at designated areas near parking areas. If you can pull yourself or your youngster away from the observation blind, continue southeast on the Kettle Lake Trail, passing between two marshes. Watch your step, as coyotes leave their fair share of scat on the trail while they hunt for the rabbits and mice that inhabit the meadow.

Kettle Lake Trail enters a woodland at 1.2 miles. The woods consist of a mix of deciduous trees a few decades old and an understory of crowded saplings and knee-high brush. The bird songs you heard in the meadow now change to songs from species that frequent woodlots, such as flycatchers and phoebes. Go slowly if you have the time and soak in the concert of chirps, peeps, and whistling runs. At 1.25 miles go left on the Multiflora Trail to loop around to the east and join the Moraine Trail, which runs north–south. At the trail junction, turn south on the Moraine Trail. (As an option, if you want to add about 0.75 mile to your hike, turn north on the Moraine Trail to arrive at the White Oak Trail, which loops through an oak forest.) But for our base hike here, follow the Moraine Trail south for nearly 0.5 mile, staying in the woods and meandering back to the starting bulletin board.

Nearby Attractions

For camping and more hiking, A. W. Marion State Park is located 4 miles southeast of Stage's Pond. The park's Hargus Lake is 145 acres of tranquility—electric boat motors only. Slide a kayak in on this lake, and for the most part you will have it all to yourself. The campground sits on a wooded ridge with 58 sites available. Call 866-644-6727 to make camping reservations.

Directions

From I-270 Exit 52, follow US 23 south 15 miles to Hagerty Road.
Turn left and drive 1.8 miles to the preserve entrance on the left.

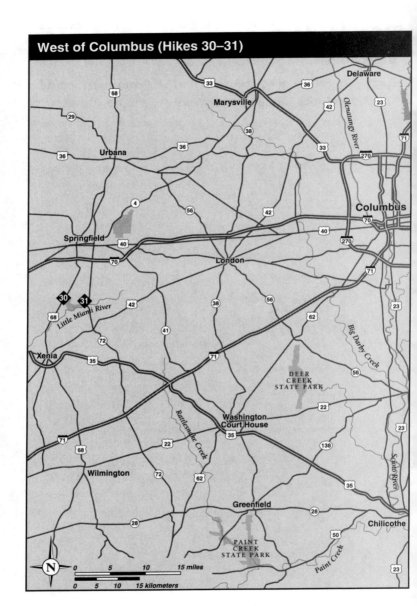

West of Columbus (Hikes 30–31)

West

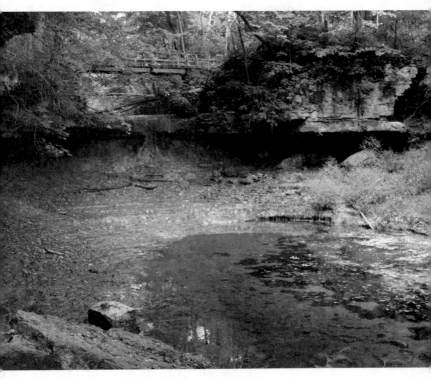

A BRIDGE CROSSES OVER THIS PICTURESQUE CASCADE.

30

Glen Helen
Nature Preserve

SCENERY: ★ ★ ★ ★ ★
TRAIL CONDITION: ★ ★
CHILDREN: ★ ★ ★
DIFFICULTY: ★ ★
SOLITUDE: ★ ★

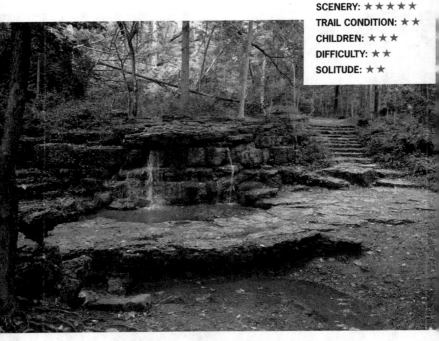

THE CALMING, FLOWING WATER OF THE YELLOW SPRING IS ALLURING.

GPS TRAILHEAD COORDINATES: N39° 48.045' W83° 53.104'

DISTANCE & CONFIGURATION: 2.3-mile loop

HIKING TIME: About 2 hours

HIGHLIGHTS: Rock formations, springs, woodlands

ELEVATION: 947' at trailhead; 983' at highest point

ACCESS: Daily, sunrise–sunset

MAPS: At nature center and **glenhelen.org**

FACILITIES: Visitor center, nature shop, raptor center, trailside museum

WHEELCHAIR ACCESS: No

COMMENTS: Pets must be on a leash; preserve rules posted at trailhead near trailside museum.

CONTACTS: 405 Corry Street, Yellow Springs, OH 45387; 937-769-1902; **glenhelen.org**

Overview

The trip begins with dozens of steps down stone stairs to a valley bottom crossed with flowing creeks. The trail rises slowly from the creek bottom to rock formations created by nature, and remnants of a man-made dam. Bypass a small waterfall and then a colorful spring emerging from stone that gave the supporting town its name—Yellow Springs. Cross a footbridge over a cascading creek and descend a forested ridge alongside a cliff edge. Do a creekside loop before re-crossing the footbridge to explore the cascading creek and returning to the starting point.

Route Details

This nature preserve covers 1,000 acres of pristine woodland valley mixed with stream life and cliff-dwelling flora and fauna. Glen Helen Nature Preserve was donated to Antioch College by an alumnus in honor of his daughter, Helen, in 1929. Its natural beauty and remarkable impressions that time has left behind are well worth the efforts to preserve it. Nature is studied here by all ages, thanks to organized programs and simple walks in the woods.

A maintained parking area ($2 fee with honor-system box) on Corry Street is where we begin. The Glen Helen Building at the north end of the parking area holds a visitor center and nature shop. You want to locate the adjacent trailside museum, which is down a pathway near the bulletin board. The entrance to the glen is located behind the museum and down a long flight of stone stairs. Doing the stairs gets the blood flowing and warms the muscles for the awaiting adventure. Once at the bottom of the stairs, a boardwalk escorts hikers to a footbridge over the 20-foot-wide Yellow Springs Creek. At this bridge, the water pools and holds fish. Use polarized sunglasses to spot the swimmers, but fishing is not allowed.

From the bridge, follow the dirt-and-pebble path east a few steps to enter the north hiking loop. It's the most popular trail in the preserve, as most of the sights are found along and around it.

Glen Helen Nature Preserve

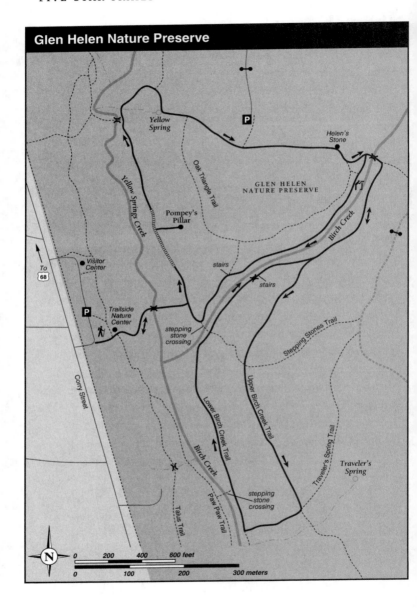

Yellow Spring

P

Helen's Stone

Oak Triangle Trail

Yellow Springs Creek

GLEN HELEN NATURE PRESERVE

Pompey's Pillar

Birch Creek

To 68

Visitor Center

stairs

stairs

P

Trailside Nature Center

stepping stone crossing

Stepping Stones Trail

Corry Street

Upper Birch Creek Trail

Lower Birch Creek Trail

Traveler's Spring Trail

Birch Creek

Traveler's Spring

Talus Trail

Paw Paw Trail

stepping stone crossing

N

0   200   400   600 feet

0   100   200   300 meters

Turn left (north) on the loop, and after traveling a couple hundred feet, you'll find a boardwalk that assists in keeping your boots dry. Another couple hundred feet beyond the start of the boardwalk is the spur trail on the right that delivers hikers to Pompey's Pillar. The short walk up to the natural rock formation is hampered by a steep slope made slick by seeping spring water. The pillar is a 15-foot-tall by 8-foot-diameter remnant of stone from the cliff wall above. Back on the main trail and 0.4 mile into the hike, the sound of falling water gets your attention. The Grotto, one of several features noted by the preserve management, is an 8-foot waterfall dropping over a small recess cave of orange and black stone. The water crosses the trail, but a flat stone footbridge elevates the path over the flowing water. A look to the opposite side of the trail brings into focus the remnants of an old dam that once created a small lake used for recreation in the early 1900s, when the preserve was a resort.

At 0.5 mile, after a bit of an uphill walk, you'll arrive at the preserve's most popular natural feature—Yellow Spring, a spring releasing iron-rich water. The water flows down a 5-foot-high stone wall and into a small pool, before following a laid stone flume and disappearing into the surrounding forest. Climb the set of stone stairs

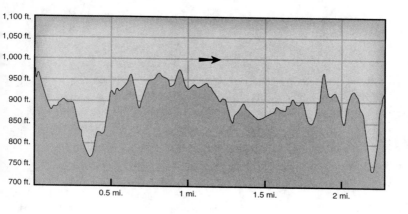

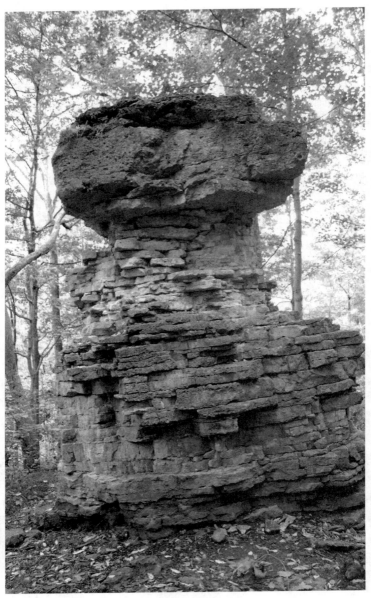

POMPEY'S PILLER, A SURVIVOR OF THOUSANDS OF YEARS OF EROSION, STANDS PROUDLY IN THE FOREST.

rising up and away from the spring to the right. The trail widens, then glides along the peak of a flat-topped ridge, but it remains under the tall forest canopy. The higher elevation lasts for only a few hundred feet before you head downhill. On the left is a huge white oak with a stone and plaque placed at the base—this is Helen's Stone. It serves as a monument to the land donor's daughter, Helen, and the place she adored. Several yards down the trail, a branch of trails spreads out. The first on the right is the Oak Triangle Trail. The second on the right is the main trail's return path to the beginning of this hike. The one to the left leads to a bridge crossing a wide creek—take this route.

Birch Creek flows under the bridge and quickly tumbles down The Cascades, pooling and then escaping and falling to the next. Exit the bridge and take the trail to the right, which follows the creek by traveling the rim of the ravine. At 0.75 mile a small path leads off to the right from the rim trail, toward the creek. Our hike will return up that trail to re-cross the bridge, but for now, stay on the current path, tiptoeing along the rim edge. Along this trek, several rocky points jut out over the ravine, offering impressive views. It's common to pass hikers while walking the main trail before the bridge, and on the north side of Birch Creek. For a better chance at nearly solitary hiking, slow the pace on the southern ridges and creek valley.

At 1 mile the rim trail you've been hiking blends into the Upper Birch Creek Trail. The smaller Stepping Stones Trail comes in from the left. Continue on Upper Birch Creek Trail until it winds down from the ridge to another intersection. At this junction take the trail to the right, which is a connector to the Lower Birch Creek Trail that parallels Yellow Springs Creek.

Follow Lower Birch Creek Trail north 0.2 mile to the confluence of Birch Creek and Yellow Springs Creek, passing a stepping-stone creek crossing on the way. A second similar crossing delivers hikers back to the north side of Birch Creek at the creek confluence. Our hike doesn't cross at either point, but continues up the south side of Birch Creek to the bridge at The Cascades. Re-cross the bridge and follow the north bank of Birch Creek back down to the creek confluence (with awesome views of the creek gorge) and turn right (north) for a few yards to exit the preserve by climbing the stone stairs you came in on.

Nearby Attractions

The town of Yellow Springs touches the western border of Glen Helen Nature Preserve. Two centuries ago, the friendly village's founders envisioned it as a utopian community. Today, the town reflects those values with a strong connection to nature and conservation. Explore various artist's studios, art galleries, and unique retail stores lining the streets, popular with kindly residents and visitors alike. John Bryan State Park is connected to Glen Helen via a hiking trail at the preserve's southeastern boundary.

Directions

From Columbus, travel I-70 west 47 miles to Exit 52. Follow US 68 south 7.6 miles to Corry Street and turn left. Drive 1,500 feet to the parking entrance on the left.

31

John Bryan State Park/ Clifton Gorge State Nature Preserve

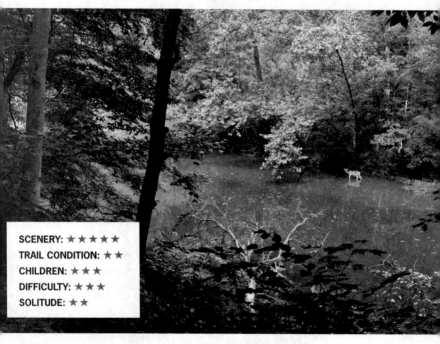

SCENERY: ★ ★ ★ ★ ★
TRAIL CONDITION: ★ ★
CHILDREN: ★ ★ ★
DIFFICULTY: ★ ★ ★
SOLITUDE: ★ ★

A DEER WADES IN THE COOL WATERS OF THE LITTLE MIAMI RIVER.

GPS TRAILHEAD COORDINATES: N39° 47.655' W83° 50.460'

DISTANCE & CONFIGURATION: 4.2-mile loop

HIKING TIME: About 3 hours

HIGHLIGHTS: Scenic river gorge, rare flora

ELEVATION: 975' at trailhead; 1,025' at highest point

ACCESS: Daily, one-half hour before sunrise to one-half hour after sunset

MAPS: At park office at John Bryan State Park entrance and **tinyurl.com/jbspmap**

FACILITIES: Latrine, drinking water, picnic shelters

WHEELCHAIR ACCESS: Limited access on Orton Memorial Trail

COMMENTS: No pets allowed at Clifton Gorge SNP; permitted at John Bryan SP if leashed.

CONTACTS: 3790 OH 370, Yellow Springs, OH 45387; 937-767-1274; **tinyurl.com/jbspark**

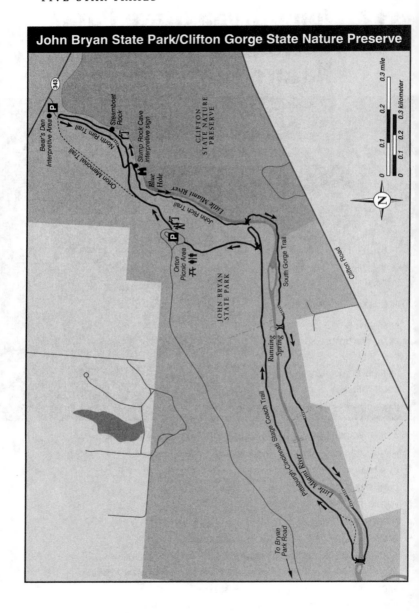

John Bryan State Park/Clifton Gorge State Nature Preserve

Overview

The Little Miami River is as scenic as they come, and fortunately, this loop explores the gorge from both sides, with two river crossings via footbridges for expanded views. The hike begins with a descent through the Clifton Gorge State Nature Preserve to the river's edge at its most rugged and gorgeous point. Return to the connecting state park by a rim trail and explore the gorge and river for 3 miles, all while trekking through one of Ohio's most beautiful parks and geological attractions.

Route Details

The scenic Little Miami River and its gorge are protected by the Clifton Gorge State Nature Preserve (visitors must abide by state nature preserve rules prohibiting the picking of vegetation and requiring hikers to stay on trail). Visitors can also explore these geological wonders on adventures at the adjoining John Bryan State Park. The 130-foot-deep Clifton Gorge was designated a National Natural Landmark in 1968, and the Little Miami River as a State and National Scenic River in 1969. Appreciation for this special place is

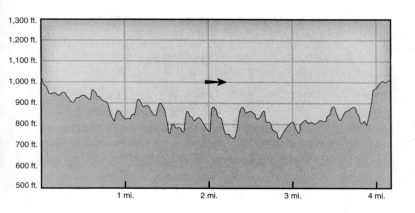

best gained by walking along the river's edge and at the base of the gorge's rock walls. When scheduling your hike, allow at least an extra hour for pausing and gazing in amazement at the gorge and its cool life-filled environment.

The Orton Picnic Area is the farthest from the park entrance, but it puts you near the border of the state nature preserve and the state park—and the trailhead of the North Rim Trail, where we begin our hike. At the picnic parking area's eastern corner, you'll find the trailhead and a plaque describing how the gorge was created and what its rock walls reveal about Ohio's geological history. Enter the forest, and a few hundred feet down the trail are two wooden observation decks on the edge of the gorge. When the trees are thick with leaves, it's difficult to see the river below from these decks. But listen closely and the sound of the Little Miami River coursing through stone can be heard no matter what the season. As you continue down the trail, be aware that the cliff edge is only a few feet away—keep yourself between a child and the edge for safety.

The trail leading down into the gorge is narrow and quite rocky and rooty. Once at the river's edge, it's easy to become mesmerized by the cool gorge atmosphere. Huge slump rocks (boulders that have fallen from cliffs above) covered with live trees and moss sit in the river and are scattered about the gorge floor. The aroma of a moist, lively river forest stirs the senses. A series of wooden walkways and decks eases the way where slump rocks and gorge walls threaten to halt a hiker's progress. The boardwalks are slippery because of the constantly moist conditions of the gorge floor. At 0.5 mile look in the middle of the river for Steamboat Rock, which was named by early visitors who saw a ship in the rock's shape—the trees growing on top are the smokestacks. The gorge is much narrower in the nature preserve than in the state park, so photographers should expect darker shooting conditions due to limited sunlight.

Just 0.2 mile upriver from Steamboat Rock, the trail leaves the gorge bottom and arrives at the top of the northern rim near the nature preserve office. A rest area called The Bear's Den Interpretive

Area welcomes hikers and offers a portable toilet, benches, and a bulletin board. The trail continues to the north and east and parallels OH 343, arriving at a parking area near Clifton Mill. Instead, our hike turns south from the rest area and follows the North Rim Trail, which delivers you back to the point where the trail led to the gorge floor. Turn right and descend to the gorge floor again, but this time turn right at the bottom and head south into John Bryan State Park. At the 1-mile point, the Blue Hole (the subject of a famous painting by Robert Duncanson) and an interpretive sign appear. The Blue Hole is a wide point in the river that also deepens, providing a calm pool. A hint of algae in the pool reflects a blue cast, which gives this favored spot on the river its name. The path at this point is known as the John Rich Trail. Watch out for the multitude of hand-sized rocks jutting up an inch or two, creating toe trippers for even agile walkers.

At 1.4 miles the nature preserve ends and the state park engulfs the entire river and provides a sturdy footbridge over the river. This point is a popular intersection for hikers, trail runners, and river explorers. Benches, trail identification signs, and a bulletin board are all found here. Cross the bridge to the south to trek the next 1.2 miles along the river to another footbridge, which you'll also cross. You're now on the South Gorge Trail, which is less traveled and maintained. A dozen small river tributaries muddy the trail. You'll cross some of the tributaries on short, rough boardwalks, but others simply have a few stones to step on, or nothing at all, so you may get dirty. The gorge gets much wider and shallower as the trail heads south, which is a plus for wildlife enthusiasts, as more habitat and space provide room to roam.

Cross the second bridge, turn back northeast, and follow the Pittsburgh-Cincinnati Stage Coach Trail. Follow this well-maintained path for about 1 mile to return to the first bridge you crossed over the river. As you hike, you will pass rock-climbing sites up the gorge to the north, which are accessible from the North Rim Trail, but out of sight of the path you're on. At the first bridge rest area, locate the trail sign on the north edge of the clearing pointing uphill to the North

Rim Trail. Work your way to the top via a narrow and extremely rocky path and turn right when you reach the North Rim Trail. Travel north on it for about 150 feet to find a small trail leading off to the left and to your vehicle at the Orton Picnic Area.

Nearby Attractions

Clifton Mill is located near the north border of Clifton Gorge State Nature Preserve, at the intersection of OH 72 and Water Street. The mill is one of the largest of its design still in existence. It's a restaurant now, but during the War of 1812 the mill processed grain to feed U.S. soldiers at war. The mill's builders took advantage of the Little Miami River as it squeezed through the beginning of the gorge, which produced higher water pressure to spin the turbine. Starting in the early 1900s, the water-powered mill also generated electricity for 30 years. Next to the mill, a 90-foot covered bridge welcomes foot traffic. Stroll across for a spectacular view of the river gorge. Glen Helen Nature Preserve neighbors John Bryan State Park.

Directions

From Columbus, travel I-70 west 47 miles to Exit 52. Follow US 68 south 6.6 miles to OH 343 and turn left at the traffic light. Go east 1 mile to OH 370 (Bryan Park Road) and turn right. Travel south 1.1 miles to the park entrance on the left. Follow the main park road to Orton Picnic Area.

Appendixes and Index

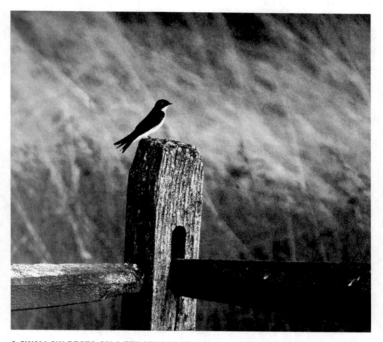

A SWALLOW RESTS ON A FENCEPOST AT PICKERINGTON PONDS METRO PARK.

Appendix A: Outdoor Retailers

CLINTONVILLE OUTFITTERS
clintonvilleoutfitters.com
2869 North High Street
Columbus, OH 43202
614-447-8902

DICK'S SPORTING GOODS
dickssportinggoods.com
1180 Polaris Parkway
Columbus, OH 43240
614-985-4729

6111 Sawmill Road
Dublin, OH 43017
614-798-1111

3700 Easton Market
Columbus, OH 43219
614-414-0200

1825 Hilliard-Rome Road
Hilliard, OH 43026
614-777-1396

1656 Stringtown Road
Grove City, OH 43123
614-801-1033

GANDER MOUNTAIN
gandermountain.com
5388 Westpointe Plaza
Columbus, OH 43228
614-921-2223

2644 Taylor Road SW
Reynoldsburg, OH 43068
614-856-0066

THE NORTH FACE
thenorthface.com
4025 Gramercy Street
Columbus, OH 43219
614-337-1147

OUTDOOR SOURCE
theoutdoorsource.com
3124 Kingsdale Center
Columbus, OH 43221
614-457-3620

5969 South Sunbury Road
Westerville, OH 43081
614-818-3620

SPORTS AUTHORITY
sportsauthority.com
6285 Sawmill Road
Dublin, OH 43017
614-799-0100

3850 Morse Road
Columbus, OH 43219
614-476-0500

5819 Chantry Drive
Columbus, OH 43232
614-860-1900

Appendix B: Places to Buy Maps

COLUMBUS METRO PARKS
metroparks.net

DELORME
delorme.com

GARMIN
garmin.com

Appendix C: Hiking Clubs

**CENTRAL OHIO HIKERS AND
BACKPACKERS**
meetup.com/Hike-COHB

**CENTRAL OHIO HIKING CLUB—
YMCA OF CENTRAL OHIO**
cohc_hikingclub@yahoo.com

HIKE OHIO
meetup.com/hiking-555

SIERRA CLUB CENTRAL OHIO GROUP
ohio.sierraclub.org/central
131 North High Street, Suite 605
Columbus, OH 43215-3026
614-461-0734

Index

About the Author

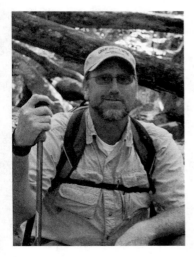

Robert Loewendick is a freelance outdoor/travel writer and guidebook author, with work regularly published in magazines, newspapers, and on the Internet. His award-winning writing has earned him active memberships in Outdoor Writers Association of America and Outdoor Writers of Ohio.

Although his passion for outdoor adventure lures him throughout the United States, Loewendick's home state of Ohio remains his favorite destination. As a young boy, he daily explored the creeks, hills, and ravines of southeast Ohio. Roaming a neighboring ridgetop with a canvas backpack purchased at an Army surplus store, loaded with a canteen of water, a peanut butter and jelly sandwich, and a self-drawn map, fueled young Loewendick's fire for adventure.

Today, Loewendick's thirst for adventure is quenched with opportunities to share with others what he regularly sees and experiences in the great outdoors. Whether it is hiking, camping, fly-fishing, kayaking, or wildlife observation, his camera and notepad are always close at hand. Inspiring youth and families to get outside more has become a cherished quest for Loewendick. He believes that if one person, especially a child, is encouraged to spend a day in the outdoors because of a story he has written or a photo he has captured, his work will have been successful.